The

Out-of-Sync

Child

Recognizing and Coping
with Sensory Processing Disorder

Revised and Updated Edition

Carol Stock Kranowitz, M.A.

A Skylight Press Book
A Perigee Book

Research about sensory processing disorder is ongoing and subject to interpretation. Although all reasonable efforts have been made to include the most up-to-date and accurate information in this book, there can be no guarantee that what we know about this complex subject won't change with time. Readers with concerns about the neurological development of their children should consult a qualified professional. Neither the publisher, the author, nor the producer take any responsibility for any possible consequences from any treatment or action by any person reading or following the information in this book.

A PERIGEE BOOK
Published by the Penguin Group
Penguin Group (USA) Inc.
375 Hudson Street, New York, New York 10014, USA
Penguin Group (Canada), 90 Eglinton Avenue East, Suite 700, Toronto, Ontario M4P 2Y3, Canada (a division of Pearson Penguin Canada Inc.)
Penguin Books Ltd., 80 Strand, London WC2R 0RL, England
Penguin Group Ireland, 25 St. Stephen's Green, Dublin 2, Ireland (a division of Penguin Books Ltd.)
Penguin Group (Australia), 250 Camberwell Road, Camberwell, Victoria 3124, Australia (a division of Pearson Australia Group Pty. Ltd.)
Penguin Books India Pvt. Ltd., 11 Community Centre, Panchsheel Park, New Delhi—110 017, India
Penguin Group (NZ), 67 Apollo Drive, Rosedale, North Shore 0632, New Zealand (a division of Pearson New Zealand Ltd.)
Penguin Books (South Africa) (Pty.) Ltd., 24 Sturdee Avenue, Rosebank, Johannesburg 2196, South Africa

Penguin Books Ltd., Registered Offices: 80 Strand, London WC2R 0RL, England

PRINTING HISTORY
ORIGINAL PERIGEE TRADE PAPERBACK EDITION / March 1998
Perigee trade paperback edition / August 2005

Perigee trade paperback ISBN: 978-0-399-53165-1

The Library of Congress has cataloged the original Perigee trade paperback as follows:

Kranowitz, Carol Stock.
    The out-of-sync child : recognizing and coping with sensory integration
dysfunction / by Carol Stock Kranowitz ;
foreword by Larry B. Silver.
    p.   cm.
    Includes bibliographical references and index.
    ISBN 0-399-52386-3
    1. Minimal brain dysfunction in children.   2. Sensorimotor integration.
3. Perceptual-motor learning.   I. Title.
RJ496.B7K72   1998
618.92'8—dc21   97-14601

PRINTED IN THE UNITED STATES OF AMERICA

20 19 18 17 16 15 14 13 12

"This book is great! It is a real contribution to the parents of the many children who are so hard to understand. It will let parents off the hook of blaming themselves . . . and will help them get on to the job of addressing the child's underlying difficulties."
—T. Berry Brazelton, MD, founder,
Brazelton Foundation, Children's Hospital, Boston

"Carol Stock Kranowitz has helped many parents understand more about [sensory processing disorder] and how it manifests itself in children."
—*Sunday News* (Lancaster, PA)

"Kranowitz writes intelligently about a bewildering topic . . . In concise, well-organized chapters, Kranowitz reveals how the tactile, vestibular (pertaining to gravity and movement), and proprioceptive (pertaining to joints, muscles, and ligaments) senses operate . . . [She] helps clear the way for families to understand a disorder that they may suspect but have not been able to pinpoint."
—*Publishers Weekly*

"A book that demystifies [sensory processing disorder]. As a music, movement, and drama teacher, [Kranowitz] has developed a purposeful curriculum that integrates sensorimotor activities into the preschool day."
—*The Ithaca Journal* (Ithaca, NY)

"Warm and wise, this book will bring both hope and practical help to parents who wonder why their kid doesn't 'fit in.' "
—Jane M. Healy, PhD, learning specialist and author of
Your Child's Growing Mind

"*The Out-of-Sync Child* does a masterful job of describing the different ways children react to sensations and integrate their responses to their world. The book provides detailed, practical information that will help parents understand how the nervous system works."
—Stanley I. Greenspan, MD, child psychiatrist and
author (with Serena Wieder) of *The Child with Special Needs*

continued . . .

"Comprehensive yet easy to understand . . . helpful tools for parents to promote healthy integration.

The Out-of-Sync Child is written for and can be easily understood by parents and non-professionals. Carol Stock Kranowitz's description and discussion of [sensory processing disorder] give a clear and concise picture of a disability. This book is a model for taking a little-known, and often-missed disability and making it accessible to the people most in need of this information.

Kranowitz gives excellent examples of typical indicators that can signal a parent (or caregiver) that a [sensory processing disorder] may be present . . . [She also] gives the reader concrete information and a testing checklist to help evaluate whether a child might have a [sensory processing disorder].

This is a great book and a must read for any parent who thinks their child might have unusual behavior difficulties. Kranowitz avoids hypertechnical language and explanations. Instead, her treatment of sensory integration issues relies on common sense and clear examples. The book is so well written that readers will be tempted to use Kranowitz's analytical approach when they read about other behavior or learning disabilities. Its calming tone and no-nonsense approach give parents the power to positively address their child's [sensory processing disorder]."

—*The Exceptional Parent*

CONTENTS

Preface by Lucy Jane Miller, PhD, OTR   *ix*
Foreword by Larry B. Silver, MD   *xiii*
Acknowledgments   *xix*
Introduction   *xxi*
How to Use This Book   *xxvii*

PART I: RECOGNIZING SENSORY PROCESSING DISORDER   1

1: *Does Your Child Have Sensory Processing Disorder?*   3
    Four Out-of-Sync Children at Home and School   4
    Sensory Processing Disorder: A Brief Definition   9
    Common Symptoms of SPD   13
    What SPD Is Not: "Look-Alike" Symptoms   21
    Associated Problems   21
    Possible Causes of SPD   37
    Who Has Sensory Processing Disorder?   38

Contents

Don't We All Experience Sensory Processing
Problems?   40
Sample Sensory-Motor History Questionnaire   40
Hope Is at Hand   47

2: *Understanding Sensory Processing—and What Can*
Go Amiss   51
   The Senses   51
   What Is Sensory Processing?   55
   The Typical Development of Sensory Processing
     in Infants and Children   66
   So, What *Is* Sensory Processing Disorder?   68
   Six Important Caveats   77
   Comparison of Typical Sensory Processing and
     Sensory Processing Disorder   79

3: *How to Tell if Your Child Has a Problem with the*
Tactile Sense   80
   Three Kindergartners at Circle Time   80
   The Smoothly Functioning Tactile Sense   82
   The Out-of-Sync Tactile Sense   84
   How the Tactile Sense Affects Everyday Skills   91
   Characteristics of Tactile Dysfunction   101

4: *How to Tell if Your Child Has a Problem with the*
Vestibular Sense   110
   Two First-Graders at the Amusement Park   110
   The Smoothly Functioning Vestibular Sense   113
   The Out-of-Sync Vestibular Sense   116
   How the Vestibular Sense Affects Everyday Skills   122
   Characteristics of Vestibular Dysfunction   129

5: *How to Tell if Your Child Has a Problem with the*
Proprioceptive Sense   134
   One Nine-Year-Old at the Swimming Pool   134
   The Smoothly Functioning Proprioceptive Sense   136

Contents

The Out-of-Sync Proprioceptive Sense 139
How the Proprioceptive Sense Affects Everyday Skills 144
Characteristics of Proprioceptive Dysfunction 148

6: *How to Tell if Your Child Has a Problem with the*
   Visual Sense 152
   Two Seventh-Graders at School 152
   The Smoothly Functioning Visual Sense 155
   The Out of-Sync Visual Sense 162
   Characteristics of Visual Dysfunction 169

7: *How to Tell if Your Child Has a Problem with the*
   Auditory Sense 174
   A Third-Grader in Music Class 174
   The Smoothly Functioning Auditory Sense 176
   The Out-of-Sync Auditory Sense 180
   Characteristics of Auditory Dysfunction 186

PART II: COPING WITH SENSORY PROCESSING DISORDER 191

8: *Diagnosis and Treatment* 193
   A Parent's Search for Answers 193
   Recognizing When Your Child Needs
      Professional Help 195
   Documenting Your Child's Behavior 198
   Diagnosing the Problem 212
   Different Therapies, Different Approaches 219
   Bringing Therapist and Child Together 225
   Keeping a Record 226

9: *Your Child at Home* 227
   A Parent's Revelation 227
   A Balanced Sensory Diet 228
   Promoting Healthy Sensory Processing at Home 231

Contents

10: *Your Child at School*   244
   What a Difference Communication Makes!   244
   If Only School Were More Like Home   245
   Deciding Whom to Tell   247
   A Good School-and-Child Match   249
   Promoting Your Child's Success at School   251

11: *Coping with Your Child's Emotions*   261
   A Typically Dreadful Morning   261
   Other Experts' Advice   263
   Dos and Don'ts for Coping   267

12: *Looking at Your Child in a New Light*   273
   A Parent's Epiphany   273
   Becoming Enlightened   274
   A Parent's Encouraging Words   279

Appendix A: The Sensory Processing Machine   283
Appendix B: Dr. Ayres's Four Levels
          of Sensory Integration   299
Glossary   305
Resources   323
About the Author   331
Selected Bibliography   333
Index   347

PREFACE TO 2ND EDITION
by Lucy Jane Miller, PhD, OTR

In 1955, Dr. A. Jean Ayres wrote her first article related to the theory of sensory integration; in 1972, her first book was published and an entire field was launched. Based on her work, Carol Kranowitz, a preschool educator for twenty-five years, helped dozens of children who manifested "sensory integration dysfunction" with the consultation of an occupational therapist (OT) who had been trained by Dr. Ayres. Dr. Ayres passed away in 1988 and with her went the knowledge base and energy that only a founder of a new vision can have. Although OTs still practiced and taught courses on sensory integration, the field had lost its leader.

In 1998, Carol published *The Out-of-Sync Child*, a book written for parents and teachers. The book was a down-to-earth explanation of: 1) the complex **theory** of sensory integration, 2) the **treatment**, called occupational therapy (OT) with a sensory integration approach, and 3) the **disorder**, now called Sensory Processing Disorder. *The Out-of-Sync Child* reenergized the world of sensory integration. Clutching Carol's book in their hands, parents came into pediatricians' and OTs' clinics, saying, "This is my child. We need occupational therapy."

Carol's goal was to write an understandable guidebook for parents whose children had sensory processing disorders. The popularity of this bestseller demonstrates both her success in achieving that goal and the urgent need for a book of this sort. *The Out-of-Sync Child* helps parents discover the missing piece in their kid's puzzle—the sensory piece. Relieved, they can see that their child's disturbing behaviors or disorganized motor abilities are related to sensory processing problems; as one parent put it, "The problem is physical, not parental."

Parents ask, "How could my child's problem have been overlooked for so long?" The answer is that few professionals, outside of OTs, knew about sensory processing disorder. When Carol's book took off, the picture changed. *The Out-of-Sync Child* is on every special needs reading list and is in the curriculum of many educational programs. It is the first book that I hand to bewildered, frustrated parents when they come to my office for answers.

Now we have the second edition of *The Out-of-Sync Child*. This resource includes updated terminology, information about children on the autistic spectrum, and new chapters on vision and hearing. The explanations of Sensory Modulation Disorder, Sensory Discrimination Disorder and Sensory-Based Motor Disorder (including dyspraxia) provide much needed clarification of the subtypes of sensory processing disorder. Carol's goal—to write for nonscientists—has remained the same. And she has succeeded again!

In this decade, I predict that we will see more scientific publications on sensory processing disorder, the inclusion of this disorder in standard diagnostic manuals, and more children getting a correct diagnosis and appropriate treatment. We will witness a generation of children with Sensory Processing Disorder grow competent and successful at home and at school. We will see OT treatment with a sensory integration approach accepted by mainstream medical and educational professionals.

Carol's contribution to the field has been immeasurable.

With her book came understanding and hope where none had been before for thousands of parents. Hope . . . and action . . . and children with brighter futures and more fulfilled lives. What could be more valuable?

Lucy Jane Miller, PhD, OTR
Associate Professor, Departments of Rehabilitation Medicine
and Pediatrics, University of Colorado Health Sciences Center

Executive Director, KID Foundation

Director, Sensory Treatment And Research
(STAR) Center
December, 2004

FOREWORD
by Larry B. Silver, MD

The brain and mind are beautifully interwoven. Our feelings, thoughts, and actions can only occur through the complex actions of the brain. Any changes in the brain, even subtle changes, can have a major impact on our feelings, thoughts, and actions. Professionals can no longer understand the psychology of the mind without understanding the biology of the brain. What is equally true is that parents of children and adolescents with modified or faulty "wiring" of the brain cannot fully understand their son or daughter without fully understanding the underlying changes in the brain and the impact these changes have on the mind.

For me, this awakening began in the 1960s. My training in Child and Adolescent Psychiatry focused only on the psychology of the mind. The explosion of brain research provided understanding of many disorders found with children and adolescents because of microscopic or chemical changes in the brain.

As we gained new knowledge about Learning Disabilities and Language Disabilities, we learned how these problems interfere with reading, writing, math, and organization skills. We learned that these problems interfere not only with academic progress, but also with success in sports, social interactions, and family life. Our growing understanding led to the fields of special education and speech-language therapy, which focus on helping individuals overcome or compensate for their disabilities.

Individuals with these changes look typical. Yet, subtle areas of their nervous systems are not functioning as they should. These changes result in behaviors that confuse, frustrate, and anger parents and teachers. They wonder why these children lack self-help skills, become aggressive or withdrawn in a group, or refuse to participate in activities or sports.

In addition to problems in learning and language, children might have problems developing the ability to process information received through their senses. These children or adolescents might have problems interpreting sights, sounds, and sensations of touch and movement. They might become unusually upset by bright lights or loud noises, or by being touched or moved unexpectedly.

They also might have problems controlling, orchestrating, and using their muscles effectively. When it is hard for them to coordinate groups of large muscles (gross motor) and/or small muscles (fine motor), they might have trouble mastering running, jumping, hopping, or climbing. They might have difficulty with buttoning, zipping, or tying, and with coloring, cutting, or writing. This difficulty getting their hands and body to do what their head is thinking creates problems with catching and throwing balls, with managing forks, pencils, and combs, and with many other essential life skills.

Dr. A. Jean Ayres studied these children with sensory and motor problems. She expanded our thinking to look at the whole integrative process needed for our brain to tell our body what to do. How does a child know how to do such complex and sequential tasks as jumping or climbing? How does a child acquire the complex skills to tie a shoe or write thoughts on the page? Dr. Ayres integrated our thinking about many sensory systems that must work independently and as a team to accomplish these and many other tasks. She described the essential roles our tactile and vestibular systems play in the process of coordinating sensory information with motor activity.

This understanding of sensory integration led to interventions to help these children. Sensory Integration Therapy focuses on correcting, improving, and/or compensating for sensory integration disorders, much as special education therapy focuses on Learning Disabilities, and speech-language therapy focuses on Language Disabilities.

We now have a greater level of understanding of these learning, language, and sensory-motor disabilities. Yet, all too often, the underlying problems are missed until the level of frustration experienced by the child or adolescent, the parents and family, and the school and teachers results in emotional, social, and family problems. Sadly, even more frequently, educational, health, and mental health professionals focus on the emotional, social, and family problems as if they were the primary issue, missing the fact that they are really secondary to underlying neurological problems.

Let me illustrate. Recently, I evaluated a four-year-old boy because his parents thought he needed to be on medication or in psychotherapy. They also asked for parent counseling to help them handle their son better. He was a "monster" at home and at nursery school. Clearly, they were overwhelmed.

His parents found themselves angry at his immature and explosive behavior. He would not dress himself, insisting that Mother dress him. He ate with his fingers. He did not play well with other children, acting bossy and insisting that they do what he wanted. No child would play with him. His favorite activity was to sit in the swing in his backyard and swing "forever."

His pediatrician told his parents to set firmer limits and to expect better behavior. His teacher was angry because he was so disruptive. He never listened to instructions and never did what he was supposed to do. The parents felt guilty that the pediatrician and teacher blamed the boy's behavior on their parenting. Yet, they did not know what else to do. Father often suggested that maybe, if Mother were more strict, their son's problems would clear up.

I was struck with how nice this child appeared when seen alone. Then, I observed him in his preschool program. In school, I could see what the teacher and parents described. He rolled around on the floor, often rolling up to another child, touching or hugging. That child would pull away, and the teacher would yell at the child I was observing.

When they had circle time, he walked around the room, refusing to sit in the circle. When playing, if another child brushed against him, he pushed the child away. I noticed how poorly he walked and ran, how clumsy he was with the blocks, and how immature his drawings were. By the end of this full-day program, he seemed tired and irritable, crying at any disappointment.

Knowing of Sensory Integration Dysfunction, I arranged for an evaluation by an occupational therapist. The underlying disabilities with motor coordination, tactile sensitivity, and vestibular insecurity were documented. Occupational therapy, not medication or psychotherapy, was started.

This child did not need to "change his behaviors." We needed to understand his behaviors and what they suggested as the probable underlying reason for the behaviors. We needed to remember that behaviors are a message, a symptom—not a diagnosis.

If professionals do not see below the surface problems and understand the underlying causes for the problems, interventions do not work. Unless the underlying problems are addressed, the emotional, social, and family problems will not improve. Our task is to not react to the behaviors with the same frustrations and feelings of failure that the child experiences. Our job is to understand the behaviors. Only with understanding can we know how to help.

As a professional who sees many children and adolescents with learning, language, and sensory integration problems, I see clearly that critical to any progress is helping parents understand the underlying neurological problems. Without their knowledge of the brain difficulties and the resulting school and life-skill problems, they cannot understand or help their son or daughter as much as they want to.

There are good books for parents on Learning Disabilities and

Language Disabilities. My frustration has been that there has not been a good book for parents on Sensory Integration Dysfunction, now known as Sensory Processing Disorder.

There is now. Carol Kranowitz has done an excellent job of taking complex material and presenting it in a way that can be understood—and used. Parents who read this book will understand motor-planning problems, as well as tactile sensitivity and vestibular-proprioceptive difficulties. The format of the book goes beyond this understanding, offering creative ideas on helping the child or adolescent handle the challenges within the family, with peers, and in school. She helps parents understand what help is needed, and how to get this help.

Knowledge is empowering, and *The Out-of-Sync Child* empowers parents to be the successful and productive parents they want to be. Thank you, Carol, for writing this book. Many families and their children will benefit.

—Larry B. Silver, MD
Clinical Professor of Psychiatry,
Georgetown University Medical Center
February, 1998

ACKNOWLEDGMENTS

Primarily, I am profoundly grateful to the late A. Jean Ayres, PhD, OTR, whom I never met but shall revere forever. Her work has touched and moved me to do all I can for children with sensory problems.

I also thank all those who made the first edition of this book possible:

Occupational therapists Lynn A. Balzer-Martin, Georgia de-Gangi, Sheri Present, Susanne Smith Roley, and Trude Turnquist.

Early childhood specialists and advocates T. Berry Brazelton, Barbara Browne, Donna Carter, Michael Castleberry, Elizabeth Dyson, Stanley Greenspan, Jane Healy, Anne Kendall, Jack Kleinmann, Patricia Lemer, Larry Silver, and Karen Strimple.

"SI parents" Chris Bridgeman, Catherine and Ron Butler, Deborah Thommasen, Linda Finkel and Vivek Talvadkar, Jacquie and Paul London, Mary Eager, and Denise McMillen.

Teachers and students at St. Columba's Nursery School in Washington, DC; Lynn Sonberg and Meg Schneider of Skylight Press; Sheila Curry Oakes, my first Perigee editor; T.J. Wylie, illustrator; and my family.

Acknowledgments

For this second edition, my everlasting love and thanks go to Lucy Jane Miller, PhD, OTR, FAOTA, who has gently guided my thinking and raised my level of understanding about sensory processing. Additionally, I thank these marvelous professionals for their wisdom and support:

Occupational therapists Marie Anzalone, Paula Aquilla, Erna Blanche, June Bunch, Anita Bundy, Sharon Cermak, Ellen Cohn, Valerie Dejean, Marie DiMatties, Winnie Dunn, Anne Fisher, Sheila Frick, Kimberly Geary, Tara Glennon, Barbara Hanft, Anne Henderson, Diana Henry, Lois Hickman, Jan Hollenbeck, Catherine Hostetler, Genevieve Jereb, Lorna Jean King, Nancy Kashman, Moya Kinnealey, Jane Koomar, Lawrene Kovalenko, Aubrey Lande, Shelly Lane, Barbara Lindner, Zoe Mailloux, Teresa May-Benson, Heather Miller-Kuhaneck, Myania Moses, Elizabeth Murray, Patricia Oetter, Beth Osten, Diane Parham, Charlane Pehoski, Norma Quirk, Sharon Ray, Judith Reisman, Eileen Richter, Roseann Schaaf, Colleen Schneck, Sherry Shellenberger, Jill Spokojny Guz, Janet Stafford, Shirley Sutton, Stacey Szklut, Sandy Wainman, Rondalyn Whitney, Julia Wilbarger, Patricia Wilbarger, Sue Wilkinson, Mary Sue Williams, and Ellen Yack.

Developmental optometrists Sanford Cohen, Kenneth Lane and Charles Shidlofsky; Nutritionist Kelly Dorfman; Physicians Fernette and Brock Eide; Psychologist Sharon Heller; Speech-language pathologists Laura Glaser, Joanne Hanson, Janet Mora and Kathleen Morris; other influential individuals including Julie Starbuck, Temple Grandin, Stephen Shore, the Pfefferle family, David Brown, Mark Zweig, and my current editor at Perigee, Marian Lizzi.

I am eternally in your debt.

—Carol Kranowitz
Bethesda, Maryland
Summer, 2005

INTRODUCTION

For twenty-five years, I taught at St. Columba's Nursery School in Washington, DC. Most preschoolers loved my classes involving music, movement, and dramatic play. Every day, small groups of three-, four-, and five-year-olds would come to my room to play, move, and learn. They happily pounded on drums and xylophones, sang and clapped, danced and twirled. They shook beanbags, manipulated puppets, and enacted fairy tales. They waved the parachute, played musical follow-the-leader games, and flowed through obstacle courses. They swooped like kites, stomped like elephants, and melted like snowmen.

Most children enjoy such activities because they have effective sensory processing—the ability to organize sensory information for use in daily life. They take in sensations of touch, movement, sight, and sound coming from their bodies and the world around them, and they respond in a well-regulated way.

Some children, however, such as Andrew, Ben, and Alice, did not enjoy coming to my classroom. Faced with the challenge of sensory-motor experiences, they became tense, unhappy, and confused. They refused to participate in the activities, or did so ineffectively, and their behavior disrupted their classmates' fun. They are the children for whom this book is written.

In my teaching career (1976–2001), I worked with more than one thousand young children. Outside of school, I taught music classes for kindergartners in my home. I choreographed children's dances for community performances. I conducted dozens of musical birthday parties. I was room mother, Cub Scout den leader, and team manager for my own sons' school and sports groups.

Many years of working with children taught me that *all* children like lively, interesting activities. They all want to join the fun—yet some don't take part. Why not? Is it that they won't—or that they can't?

When I began teaching, the nonparticipants puzzled me. Why, I wondered, were these children so difficult to reach? Why did they fall apart when it was time to join the fun?

Why did Andrew buzz around the room's perimeter while his classmates, sitting on the rug, sang "The Wheels on the Bus"?

Why did Ben tap, tap, tap his shoulders when the musical instructions were to tap, tap, tap his knees?

Why did Alice flop onto her stomach, "too tired" to sit up and strike together two rhythm sticks?

At first, these children annoyed me. They made me feel like a bad teacher. They also made me feel like a bad person when their inattention or disruptive behavior caused me to react negatively. Indeed, on one regrettable occasion, I told a child that turning away and covering his ears when I played the guitar was "just plain rude." That day I went home and wept.

Every evening, while preparing dinner or engaging with my own sons, I would muse about these students. I couldn't get a handle on them. They had no identified special needs. They weren't unloved or disadvantaged. Some seemed to misbehave on purpose, like sticking a foot out to trip a classmate, while others seemed to move without any purpose at all, in an aimless or listless manner. Little about their behavior could be classified, except for a shared inability to enjoy the activities that children traditionally relish.

I wasn't the only one who was stumped. Karen Strimple,

director of St. Columba's Nursery School, and the other teachers were equally puzzled by the same children. The children's parents were often concerned, especially when they compared their child's behavior with that of their other, more "together" offspring. And, if caring parents and teachers were frustrated, how must the children themselves feel?

They felt like failures.

And we teachers felt that we were failing them.

We knew we could do better. After all, since the 1970s, St. Columba's had been mainstreaming into its regular school program a number of children with identified special needs. We were extremely successful with these children. Why were we less successful teaching certain "regular" kids with subtle, unidentified problems? We wanted an answer.

The answer came from Lynn A. Balzer-Martin, PhD, OTR, a St. Columba's parent and a pediatric occupational therapist. Since the 1970s, Lynn had been an educational consultant for our mainstreaming program—called Inclusion today. Her primary work, however, was diagnosing and treating young children who had academic and behavior problems stemming from a neurological inefficiency—then called Sensory Integration Dysfunction.

An occupational therapist, A. Jean Ayres, PhD, was the pioneer who first described the problem. About fifty years ago, Dr. Ayres formulated a theory of Sensory Integration Dysfunction and led other occupational therapists in developing intervention strategies. Her book, *Sensory Integration and the Child*, presents a thorough explanation of this misunderstood problem and is required reading for anyone interested in grasping its technicalities.

Sensory Integration Dysfunction, now known as Sensory Processing Disorder (SPD), is not a new problem. It is a new definition of an old problem.

SPD can cause a bewildering variety of symptoms. When their central nervous systems are ineffective in processing sensory information, children have a hard time functioning in daily life. They may look fine and have superior intelligence, but may be awkward and clumsy, fearful and withdrawn, or hostile and aggressive. SPD can affect not only how they move and learn, but also how they behave, how they play and make friends, and especially how they feel about themselves.

Many parents, educators, doctors, and mental health professionals have difficulty recognizing SPD. When they don't recognize the problem, they may mistake a child's behavior, low self-esteem, or reluctance to participate in ordinary childhood experiences for hyperactivity, learning disabilities, or emotional problems. Unless they are educated about SPD, few people understand that bewildering behavior may stem from a poorly functioning nervous system.

Dr. Lynn Balzer-Martin, like other students of Dr. Ayres's work, was trained to recognize and treat sensory problems. Her growing concern was that many of her clients were not sent to her for a diagnosis until well after they had run into trouble at school or at home, at the ages of six, seven, or eight. She was anxious to identify children at younger ages because the brain is most receptive to change while it is developing.

Preschoolers, whose nervous systems are still developing rapidly, stand a good chance to benefit from therapeutic intervention. Lynn knew that if SPD could be detected in three-, four-, or five-year-olds, these children could receive individualized treatment that would prevent later social and academic impasses.

The challenge was to find a way to identify preschoolers with SPD, because the available standardized tests are inappropriate for the "little guys." Lynn conceived of a quick, effective screening to see whether very young children had the neurological foundations necessary for developing into well-organized people. She asked us if we were interested.

Were we interested?!

Thus, everything came together at once. We wanted to learn more about our worrisome students. Lynn wanted to try out her screening idea. The Katharine P. Maddux Foundation, which already funded our flagship mainstreaming program, was urging us to develop more projects designed to improve the physical, mental, and emotional health of children and their families.

Lynn's first goal was to educate us about sensory processing and then, with our help, to devise a screening program that would be developmentally suitable for preschoolers.

The screening process would be fun for the children. It would be simple enough for many schools to duplicate. It would be short, yet thorough enough to enable educators to distinguish between basic immaturity and possible SPD in young children.

Most important, it would provide data that would encourage parents to seek early intervention for their children with an appropriate professional (such as an occupational therapist, physical therapist, or sometimes a psychologist or speech/language pathologist). The purpose of early intervention is to help children function better—even beautifully—in their classrooms, in their homes, and in their daily lives.

In 1987, with the support of the school community and with my eager assistance, Lynn instituted a program at St. Columba's in which all 130 students undergo an annual screening. We began to guide identified children into early intervention therapy. And we began to see immediate, positive, exhilarating results as these children's skills began to improve.

Under Lynn's guidance, I studied and learned everything I could about the subject. I learned to screen the children and to compile data gleaned from teachers, parents, and direct observations. I learned to make sense of some children's mystifying behavior.

As my knowledge increased, so did my teaching skills. I learned to help my co-teachers understand why these children marched to a different drummer. I gave workshops at other preschools and elementary schools to train educators to recognize signs of this subtle problem. I added activities in my class that promote healthy sensory-motor development for *all* children.

I rejoiced in the strides that children such as Andrew, Ben, and Alice made soon after they began occupational therapy. Incredibly, as they acquired more efficient sensory-motor skills, they relaxed, became more focused, and began to enjoy school. Now, when I went home at the end of the day, it wasn't to weep—it was to celebrate!

While my expertise grew, I learned that explaining SPD to parents requires time and skill. When children who were screened showed clear evidence of dysfunction, Karen and I asked their parents to come in to observe them in the classroom and on the playground. Then we would sit down for a private conference to discuss our observations.

In these conferences, we described Sensory Processing Disorder and why we suspected it as a cause of their child's difficulties. We explained that the problem is treatable. We said that while older children and even adults can improve with treatment, early intervention produces the most dramatic results. We tried to allay parents' fears, assuring them that SPD did not suggest that their child was mentally deficient, or that they were inadequate parents.

We understood that this information inevitably filled parents with anxiety, questions, and misapprehensions. Often, they dashed to their pediatrician, who, unfamiliar with SPD, mistakenly dismissed it as a problem that the child would outgrow.

We knew that we raised more questions than it was possible to answer in a half-hour conference.

Thus, this book was conceived to explain sensory processing and its counterpart, Sensory Processing Disorder, to parents, teachers, and other non-OTs who are new at this. This second edition, seven years after the first, contains up-to-date information that may also help those who are already experienced in caring for children with other, more observable disabilities, many of which overlap with SPD.

I have attempted to make the explanations reader-friendly. They will remind you of or introduce you to terms that early childhood professionals commonly use—terms with which you need to be familiar.

The viewpoint is "teacherly" and may differ here and there from other clinical or research-oriented points-of-view. Understanding SPD from different perspectives will allow you to understand your child (or student) better, and that is the book's most important purpose. Then you will be prepared to provide the help the child needs to become as competent and confident as possible.

HOW TO USE THIS BOOK

Whether or not your child has been diagnosed, this book will help you understand and cope with Sensory Processing Disorder (SPD), also known as Sensory Integration Dysfunction. The book is not just for parents. It is also for teachers, medical doctors, occupational therapists, psychologists, grandparents, baby-sitters, and others who care for the out-of-sync child.

As a teacher, I have witnessed how SPD plays out. I have seen behavior that parents, pediatricians, and even therapists don't have the chance to observe. Thus, the book, written from a teacher's perspective, offers insights that a specialist in another field of child development might overlook.

Part I includes an overview of SPD and how it affects children's behavior; checklists and a questionnaire (for you to mark) of symptoms, associated problems, and characteristics of out-of-sync children; a guide to typical neurological development; how the fundamental senses work, how they influence everyday life, and what happens when they're inefficient; anecdotes contrasting the responses of children with and without efficient sensory processing; and the hope that a solution to your child's difficulties is at hand.

Part II includes criteria and guidance for getting a diagnosis and treatment; examples of charts for documenting your child's behavior; tips for keeping a running record; how occupational therapy helps, and a look at other therapies; suggestions for a balanced "sensory diet" and for improving your young child's skills at home; ideas to share with teachers for helping your child at school; coping techniques to handle your child's emotions and to improve family life; and encouragement and support—for you and your child are not alone!

The Out-of-Sync Child concludes with two Appendices—The Sensory Processing Machine, to explain the role of the central nervous system, and Dr. Ayres' Four Levels of Sensory Integration; Resources for materials and support; a Selected Bibliography; and a Glossary and Index.

Read the book cover to cover to get a broad picture of Sensory Processing Disorder. Use it as a reference to refresh yourself on a specific area of dysfunction. With pencil in hand, use it as a workbook. Keep it handy as an activity book. Use it to learn about your child—and perhaps to learn about yourself, as well.

Part I

Recognizing

Sensory

Processing

Disorder

Chapter One

DOES YOUR CHILD HAVE SENSORY PROCESSING DISORDER?

Surely, you know a child who is oversensitive, clumsy, picky, fidgety, and out of sync. That child may be your son or daughter, your student or Scout, your nephew or neighbor . . . or the child you were, once upon a time. That child may have Sensory Processing Disorder (SPD), a common, but misunderstood, problem that affects children's behavior, influencing the way they learn, move, relate to others, and feel about themselves.

To illustrate how sensory processing problems play out, the stories of four out-of-sync children and the parents struggling to raise them are presented in the next pages. You will also see lists of common symptoms, associated problems, and possible causes.

This information will help you determine whether SPD affects your child. If your child has a significant problem, the information may strike you like a bolt of lightning. You may instantly recognize the signs and be relieved to have some answers, at last. Even if your child has a mild problem, you can use this information to gain new insight into his or her puzzling behavior.

Whether SPD is major or minor, the child who is out of sync

needs understanding and help, for no child can overcome the obstacles alone.

FOUR OUT-OF-SYNC CHILDREN
AT HOME AND SCHOOL

Tommy is the only son of two adoring parents. They waited a long time before having a child and rejoiced in his arrival. And when they finally got him in their hands, they got a handful.

The day after he was born, his parents were told that he could not stay in the hospital nursery because his wailing disturbed the other infants. Once he arrived home, he rarely slept through the night. Although he nursed well and grew rapidly, he adamantly rejected the introduction of solid food and vigorously resisted being weaned. He was a very fussy baby.

Today, Tommy is a fussy three-year-old. He is crying because his shoes are too tight, his socks too lumpy. He yanks them off and hurls them away.

To prevent a tantrum, his mother lets him wear bedroom slippers to school. She has learned that if it isn't shoes and socks that bother him, it's inevitably something else that will trip him up during the day.

His parents bend over backwards, but pleasing their healthy, attractive child is a challenge. Everything scares him or makes him miserable. His response to the world is, "Oh, no!" He hates the playground, the beach, and the bathtub. He refuses to wear hats or mittens, even on the coldest days. Getting him to eat is a trial.

Arranging play dates with other children is a nightmare. Going to the barber shop is a disaster. Wherever they go, people turn away—or stare.

His teacher reports that he avoids painting and other messy activities. He fidgets at story time and doesn't pay attention. He lashes out at his classmates for no apparent reason. He is, however, the world's best block builder, as long as he isn't crowded.

Tommy's pediatrician tells his parents nothing is wrong with him, so they should stop worrying and just let him grow. His grandparents say he's spoiled and needs stricter discipline. Friends suggest going on a vacation without him.

Tommy's parents wonder if yielding to his whims is wise, but it's the only method that works. They are exhausted, frustrated, and stressed. They can't understand what makes him tick.

Sweet Vicki, a pudgy first-grader, is often in a daze. Her response to the world buzzing around her seems to be, "Ho, hum." She doesn't seem to see where she is going, so she bumps into furniture and stumbles on grass. When she tumbles, she is slow to extend her foot or hand to break the fall. She doesn't appear to hear ordinary sounds, either. Other six-year-olds may have developed the sense to stop, look, and listen, but not Vicki. She disregards important sensory information coming at her from all sides.

In addition, Vicki fatigues easily. A family outing or trip to the playground quickly wears her out. She sighs, "You go. I don't want to. I'm too pooped."

Because of her lethargy, her parents find that getting her out of bed, asking her to put on her coat, or maneuvering her into the car is an ordeal. She takes a long time to carry out simple, familiar movements. In every situation, it is as if she is saying, "Huh? How am I supposed to do this?"

Nonetheless, she wants to be a ballerina when she grows up. Every day she sprawls in front of the TV to watch her favorite video, *The Nutcracker*. When her beloved Sugar Plum Fairies begin to dance, she hauls herself to a stand to sway along with them. Her movements, however, do not match the musical rhythm or tempo. Ear-body coordination is not her forte.

Vicki begged for ballet lessons, but they have not been going well. She loves her purple tutu but cannot differentiate top from bottom and needs help to get into it. Once attired in tulle, tiara, and slippers, she plops down. She has no idea how to bend her knees in a plié or stretch her leg in an arabesque. At dancing school,

Vicki usually gets cold feet and clings like taffy to her mother's leg.

Vicki's parents disagree on the best way to handle her. Her father picks her up and put her places—in bed, in the car, on a chair. He also dresses her, as she has trouble orienting her limbs to get into her clothes. He refers to her as his "little noodle."

Vicki's mother, on the other hand, believes Vicki will never learn to move with confidence, much less become a ballerina, if she doesn't learn independence. Her mother says, "I think she would stick to one spot all day if I let her."

Although Vicki lacks "oomph" and is definitely not a self-starter, certain kinds of movement will get her on her toes. She becomes livelier after getting into unusual positions—rocking forward and back while on all fours, hanging over the edge of her bed upside down, and swinging on her tummy. She still has not figured out how to pump. She loves to be pushed for a long time on the playground swing—and when she stops, she is never dizzy, as other children might be.

Being pushed *passively* arouses Vicki, as does *actively* pushing something heavy. Occasionally, Vicki crams books into her doll carriage and shoves it around the house. She volunteers to push the grocery cart and carry bags into the house. She also enjoys pulling her big sister in a wagon. After pushing and pulling weighty loads, she has some energy for half an hour or so and then sinks back into her customary lethargy.

At school, Vicki mostly sits. Her teacher says, "Vicki has difficulty socializing and getting involved in classroom activities. It's like her batteries are low. She needs a jump start just to get going. Then she loses interest and gives up easily."

Vicki's behavior mystifies her parents. Their experiences with their two other active children have not prepared them to deal with her atypical behavior.

Paul is an extremely shy nine-year-old. He also moves awkwardly, has poor posture and balance, and falls frequently. He does not have the know-how to play, and when he's in a group with other children, usually he watches dolefully or shuffles away. At their grandparents' house one Sunday afternoon, Paul's twelve-year-old cousin, Prescott, invites Paul to play marbles and shoot baskets with him. Paul gives the activities a half-hearted try, shrugs and turns away. "I can't do that," he says. "Anyway, what's the point?"

Paul dislikes school. Sometimes he asks to stay home, and his parents let him. He says he doesn't want to go to school because he's no good at anything, and everyone laughs at him.

Paul's teacher notes that he has a long attention span and an above-average reading ability. She wonders why a child with so much information to share becomes paralyzed when he has to write a paper. True, his handwriting is laborious, and his papers are crumpled and full of erasure holes. True, he has a "death grip" on pencils, fixes his elbow to his ribs, and sticks his tongue out when he writes. True, he often slips off the chair when he is concentrating hard on written work. His handwriting skills, she hopes, will improve with more practice. She says he just needs to get organized so he can pay more attention to his assignments and do neater work.

His parents wonder why he is a misfit at school, because he has always fit right into their sedate lifestyle. Paul is a modest child, rarely seeking attention. He can spend hours slumped over his baseball cards, completely self-absorbed.

Paul's parents think he is the perfect child. They observe that he is unlike other kids, who are loud and mischievous. He never makes trouble, although he is somewhat clumsy, often dropping dishes and breaking toys that require simple manipulation. But then, his parents are somewhat clumsy, too, and have come to believe that physical prowess is unimportant. They are glad that their son is quiet, well-mannered and bookish, just like them.

Something, however, is getting in his way. His parents have no idea what.

Sebastian, eight, fidgets constantly. At school, he riffles book pages, twiddles with markers, taps rulers and breaks pencils. He clicks his teeth and chews his collar.

Sebastian's knees bounce, his feet tap, his eyes dart, his fingers flap his earlobes. He tips his desk chair way back and then brings it forward with a jolt. He squirms in his seat, sitting on his feet or squeezing his knees to his chest. He jumps out of his seat every chance he gets to sharpen his pencil or pitch a wadded paper toward the wastebasket.

His nonstop activity distracts his classmates and teacher. He used to twirl the lanyard with his latchkey around his finger. Once he let go accidentally and it whirled across the room and hit the blackboard. Now he hands the lanyard over to his teacher every morning so it won't annoy or hurt anyone.

Sebastian seeks sensations: "More, more, more!" He is the child who "gotta touch," even when it should be clear that touching is inappropriate.

One day the teacher is preparing a science lesson. She lays out white glue, laundry borax, and water—the ingredients to make a pliable substance called "Stretchy Gook." Sebastian is interested and hovers nearby, twitching his fingers and hopping from foot to foot. The teacher says, "Please don't touch a thing until the other kids join us," but he reaches forward and knocks over the bottle of glue, spilling it across the table.

"Sebastian! You did it again!" the teacher says.

"I didn't mean to!" Sebastian cries. He shakes his head vigorously from side to side and jumps up and down. "Oh," he moans, "why do I always get in trouble?"

"Oh," moans the teacher, mopping up the mess, "what shall I do with you?"

Why are Tommy, Vicki, Paul, and Sebastian out of sync? Their parents, teachers, and pediatricians don't know what to think.

The children have no identified disabilities, such as cerebral palsy or impaired eyesight. They seem to have everything going for them: They're healthy, intelligent, and dearly loved. Yet they struggle with the basic skills of managing their responses to ordinary sensations, of planning and organizing their actions, and of regulating their attention and activity levels.

Their common problem is Sensory Processing Disorder.

SENSORY PROCESSING DISORDER:
A BRIEF DEFINITION

Sensory Processing Disorder (SPD) is the inability to use information received through the senses in order to function smoothly in daily life. SPD is not one specific disorder, as blindness or deafness is, but rather an umbrella term to cover a variety of neurological disabilities. SPD is also called Sensory Integration Dysfunction (SI Dysfunction) and Dysfunction in Sensory Integration (DSI). Chapter Two explains SPD in more depth.

The late A. Jean Ayres, PhD, an occupational therapist, was the first to describe sensory problems as the result of inefficient neurological processing. In the 1950s and 1960s, she developed a theory of sensory integration and taught other occupational therapists how to assess it.

Many brilliant occupational therapists—Dr. Ayres' colleagues and disciples—have continued her work. Over the decades, as other health professionals, parents and educators have become attuned to the subject, some terminology has been confused, misused, or used in conflicting ways.

For example, you may hear a pediatrician remark, "I believe your child has some SI," or a mother says, "My child has SI." The response to those comments is, "Great! SI (sensory integration) is what we all want!" What the doctor and parent mean is, "The child has sensory integration *problems*."

Using inconsistent terminology hurts the child when therapists, doctors, parents, and insurance companies misunderstand one another and disagree on appropriate treatment. In 2004, a group led by Lucy Jane Miller, PhD, including Sharon Cermak, EdD, Shelly Lane, PhD, and Marie Anzalone, ScD, with Beth Osten and Stanley Greenspan, MD, proposed to clarify the terminology so that all parties are in sync when discussing a person with sensory difficulties.

Using Dr. Ayres' original concepts, Dr. Miller's committee classified the diagnostic groups of SPD in an updated version. In this classification, Sensory Processing Disorder is the overall term, encompassing three main categories (Sensory Modulation Disorder, Sensory Discrimination Disorder, and Sensory-Based Motor Disorder) and their subtypes.

Categories and Subtypes of Sensory Processing Disorder

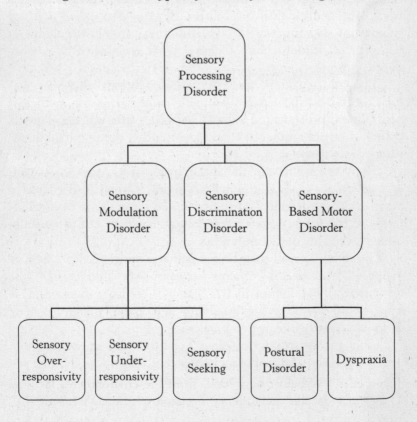

The revisions in this second edition of *The Out-of-Sync Child* reflect Dr. Miller's work. Her upcoming book, *Sensational Children: Hope and Help for Children with Sensory Processing Disorder* (Putnam, 2006), explains the terminology in detail.

SPD happens in the central nervous system, at the "head" of which is the brain. When processing is disorderly, the brain cannot do its most important job of organizing sensory messages. The child cannot respond to sensory information to behave in a meaningful, consistent way. He may also have difficulty using sensory information to plan and carry out actions that he needs to do. Thus, he may not learn easily.

Learning is a broad term. One kind of learning is called adaptive behavior, which is the ability to change one's behavior in response to new circumstances, such as learning to meet different teachers' expectations. Adaptive behavior—or adaptive responses—is goal directed and purposeful.

Another kind of learning is motor learning, which is the ability to develop increasingly complex movement skills after one has mastered simpler ones. Examples are learning to use a pencil after learning to use a crayon, or learning to catch a ball after learning to throw one.

A third kind of learning is academic learning. This is the ability to acquire conceptual skills, such as reading, computing, and applying what one learns today to what one learned yesterday.

HOW INEFFICIENT SENSORY PROCESSING LEADS TO INEFFICIENT LEARNING

Your child yanks the cat's tail, and the cat hisses, arches its back, and spits. Normally, through experience, a child will learn not to repeat such a scary experience. He learns to be cautious. In the future, his behavior will be more adaptive.

The child with SPD, however, may have difficulty "reading cues," verbal or nonverbal, from the environment. He may not decode the auditory message of the cat's hostile hissing, the visual message of the cat's arched back, or the tactile message of spit on his cheek. He misses the "big picture," and may not learn appropriate caution.

Or the child can read the cat's reaction, but is unable to change his behavior and stop himself. He receives the sensory information, but can't organize it to respond efficiently.

Or the child sometimes can take in sensations, organize them, and respond appropriately—but not today. This may be one of his "off" days.

Possible results:

• The child may never learn and may get repeatedly scratched. Thus, he may continue this risky behavior until someone removes the cat, or the cat learns to avoid the child. The child loses a chance to learn how to relate positively to other living creatures.

• The child becomes fearful of the cat. He may not understand cause and effect and may be bewildered by what seems to be unpredictable cat behavior. He may become afraid of other animals, too.

• Eventually, the child may learn about cause and effect, may learn to grade his movements, may learn to treat animals gently, and may grow up to love cats—but this will happen only with much conscious effort, after much time and many, many scratches.

The brain-behavior connection is very strong. Because the child with SPD has a disorganized brain, many aspects of his behavior are disorganized. His overall development is disorderly and his participation in childhood experiences is spotty, reluctant or inept. For the out-of-sync child, performing ordinary tasks and responding to everyday events can be enormously challenging.

The inability to function smoothly is not because the child won't, but because he can't.

COMMON SYMPTOMS OF SPD

Below are four checklists of common symptoms of SPD. The first list, "Sensory Modulation Problems," pertains to how a child regulates his responses to sensations. Some children with poor modulation are primarily overresponsive, some are primarily underresponsive, some are primarily sensory seeking, and others fluctuate.

The second list, "Sensory Discrimination Problems," includes examples of how a child may have difficulty in distinguishing one sensation from another.

The third list, "Sensory-Based Motor Problems," has examples of how a child may position his body in unusual ways and have difficulty in conceiving of an action to do, planning how to organize and move his body, and carrying out the plan.

The fourth list, "Associated Regulatory and Behavior Problems," pertains to issues that can result from inefficient sensory processing as well as from other developmental problems. The child with these problems does not necessarily have SPD.

As you check the symptoms that you recognize, please understand that they will vary from child to child, because every brain is unique (just as every fingerprint is unique). No child will exhibit all the symptoms. Still, if several descriptions fit your own son or daughter, chances are that he or she has some degree of SPD.

The child with severe SPD shows many symptoms. Interacting with other people, functioning in daily life, and succeeding in the occupation of being a child are greatly impaired. The child with mild SPD is slightly impaired and may find ways to compensate—but the problem is frequently overlooked. The child with moderate SPD is somewhere in between.

Whether the child has severe, moderate or mild dysfunction, he or she needs understanding and help. Ignoring problems will not make them disappear.

Sensory Modulation Problems

The first and most common category of SPD is Sensory Modulation Disorder. This is suspected when the child exhibits one or more symptoms with frequency, intensity and duration. Frequency means several times a day. Intensity means that he adamantly avoids sensory stimulation, or throws his whole body and soul into getting the stimulation he needs. Duration means that this unusual response lasts for several minutes or longer.

These charts will give you a quick overview of common problems. Later chapters will provide more details.

Sensations	Overresponsive Child ("Oh, no!")	Underresponsive Child ("Ho, hum.")	Sensory-Seeking Child ("More!")
Touch	☐ Avoids touching or being touched by objects and people. Reacts with a fight-or-flight response to getting dirty, to certain textures of clothing and food, and to light, unexpected, touch.	☐ Is unaware of messy face, hands, or clothes, and may not know whether she has been touched. Does not notice how things feel and often drops items. Lacks "inner drive" to handle toys.	☐ Wallows in mud, dumps out bins of toys and rummages through them purposelessly, chews on inedible objects such as shirt cuffs, rubs against walls and furniture, and bumps into people.

14

Sensations	Overresponsive Child ("Oh, no!")	Underresponsive Child ("Ho, hum.")	Sensory-Seeking Child ("More!")
Movement and Balance	☐ Avoids moving or being unexpectedly moved. Is insecure and anxious about falling or being off balance. Keeps feet on the ground. Gets carsick.	☐ Does not notice or object to being moved. Is unaware of falling and protects self poorly. Usually is not a self-starter, but once started, swings for a long time without getting dizzy.	☐ Craves fast and spinning movement, and may not get dizzy. Moves constantly, fidgets, gets into upside-down positions, is a dare-devil, and takes bold risks.
Body Position and Muscle Control	☐ May be rigid and uncoordinated. Avoids playground activities that bring strong sensory input to muscles.	☐ Lacks inner drive to move for play. Becomes more alert after actively pushing, pulling, lifting, and carrying heavy loads.	☐ Craves bear hugs and being squeezed and pressed. Seeks heavy work and more vigorous playground activities than others.

While difficulties with touch, movement and body position are the telltale signs of SPD, the child may also respond in atypical ways to sights, sound, smells, and tastes:

Sensations	Overresponsive Child ("Oh, no!")	Underresponsive Child ("Ho, hum.")	Sensory-Seeking Child ("More!")
Sights	☐ Gets overexcited with too much to look at (words, toys, or	☐ Ignores novel visual stimuli, e.g., obstacles in her path.	☐ Seeks visually stimulating scenes and screens for lengthy times.

Sensations	Overresponsive Child ("Oh, no!")	Underresponsive Child ("Ho, hum.")	Sensory-Seeking Child ("More!")
	people). Covers eyes, has poor eye contact, is inattentive to desk work, over-reacts to bright light. Is ever alert and watchful.	Responds slowly to approaching objects. May not turn away from bright light. Stares at and looks right through faces and objects.	Is attracted to shiny, spinning objects and bright, flickering light, such as strobe lights or sunlight streaming through blinds.
Sounds	☐ Covers ears to close out sounds or voices. Complains about noises, such as vacuum clean-ers, that don't bother others.	☐ Ignores ordi-nary sounds and voices, but may "turn on" to exag-gerated musical beats or extremely loud, close, or sudden sounds.	☐ Welcomes loud noises and TV volume. Loves crowds and places with noisy action. May speak in a booming voice.
Smells	☐ Objects to odors, such as a ripe banana, that others do not notice.	☐ May be un-aware of un-pleasant odors and unable to smell his meal.	☐ Seeks strong odors, even objec-tionable ones, and sniffs food, people, and objects.
Tastes	☐ Strongly ob-jects to certain textures and temperatures of foods. May frequently gag while eating.	☐ May be able to eat very spicy food without reaction.	☐ May lick or taste inedible objects, like Play-Doh and toys. May prefer very spicy or very hot foods.

Sensory Discrimination Problems

Another category of Sensory Processing Disorder is Sensory Discrimination Disorder, which is the difficulty in distinguishing one sensation from another, or in understanding what a sensation means. The child with poor discrimination may have a problem protecting himself or learning something new. Often, he also is underresponsive and has a Sensory-Based Motor Disorder.

Sensations	Child with Sensory Discrimination Disorder ("Huh?")
Touch	☐ Cannot tell where on her body she has been touched. Has poor body awareness and is "out of touch" with her hands and feet. Cannot distinguish objects by feel alone (without seeing). Is a sloppy dresser and unusually awkward with buttons, barrettes, etc. Handles eating utensils and classroom tools inefficiently. May also have difficulty processing sensations of pain and temperature, e.g., gauging how serious a bruise is and whether pain is better or worse, or whether she is hot or cold.
Movement and Balance	☐ Cannot feel himself falling, especially when eyes are closed. Becomes easily confused when turning, changing directions, or getting into a stance where his head is outside an upright, two-footed position. May be unable to tell when he has had enough movement.
Body Position and Muscle Control	☐ May be unfamiliar with own body, lacking "internal eyes." Is "klutzy" and has difficulty positioning limbs for getting dressed or pedaling a bike. Cannot grade movements smoothly, using too much or not enough force for handling pencils and toys or for pushing open doors and kicking balls. May bump, crash, and "dive bomb" into others in interactions.

Sensations	Child with Sensory Discrimination Disorder ("Huh?")
Sights	☐ If problem is caused by SPD (and not nearsightedness, for example), may confuse likenesses and differences in pictures, written words, objects, and faces. In social interactions, may miss people's expressions and gestures. Has difficulty with visual tasks, such as lining up columns of numbers or judging where things are in space— himself, included—and how to move to avoid bumping into objects.
Sounds	☐ If problem is caused by SPD (and not ear infections or dyslexia, for example), may have difficulty recognizing the differences between sounds, especially consonants at ends of words. Cannot repeat or make up rhymes. Sings out of tune. Looks to others for cues, as verbal instructions may be confusing. Has poor auditory skills, such as picking out a teacher's voice from a noisy background, or paying attention to one sound without being distracted by other sounds.
Smell and Tastes	☐ Cannot distinguish distinct smells such as lemons, vinegar, or soap. Cannot distinguish tastes or tell when food is too spicy, salty, or sweet. May choose or reject food based on the way it looks.

Sensory-Based Motor Problems

The third category of SPD is Sensory-Based Motor Disorder, which includes two types. One type is Postural Disorder, involving problems with movement patterns, balance and using both sides of the body together (bilateral coordination). The problem often coexists with underresponsivity and poor sensory discrimination.

Sensory-Based Motor Skills	Child with Postural Disorder ("Don't want to.")
Components of Movement	☐ May be tense or have "loose and floppy" muscle tone, a weak grasp on objects, and difficulty getting into and maintaining a stable position. Has a problem fully flexing and extending her limbs. Slouches and sprawls. Has difficulty shifting weight to crawl and rotating body to throw a ball.
Balance	☐ Loses balance easily when walking or changing positions. Trips on air.
Bilateral Coordination	☐ Has difficulty using both sides of the body together for jumping symmetrically, catching balls, clapping, holding swing chains, and pumping. Has difficulty using one hand to assist the other, such as holding a paper while cutting, or a cup while pouring.
Unilateral Coordination	☐ May not have a definite hand preference. May use either hand to reach for an object or to use tools such as pens and forks. May switch object from right to left hand when handling it, eat with one hand but draw with the other, or manipulate scissors using both hands.
Crossing the Midline	☐ May have difficulty using a hand, foot, or eye on the opposite side of the body, such as using one hand to paint or reading a line across a paper.

The second type of Sensory-Based Motor Disorder is Dyspraxia, or difficulty with praxis (Greek for "doing, action, practice"). Praxis is based on unconscious sensory processing as well as conscious thought. The dyspraxic child has problems performing coordinated and voluntary actions.

Sensory-Based Motor Skills	Child with Dyspraxia ("I can't do that.")
Components of Praxis	☐ May have difficulty: 1) conceiving of a new, complex action to do, 2) sequencing the steps and organizing body movements to do it, and 3) carrying out the multiple-step motor plan. May be awkward, clumsy, apparently careless (even when trying to be careful) and accident prone.
Gross-Motor Planning	☐ May have poor motor coordination and be clumsy when moving around furniture, in a crowded room or on a busy playground. Has problem with stairs, obstacle courses, playground equipment, and large-muscle activities such as walking, marching, crawling, and rolling. Ability to learn new motor skills, such as skipping, may develop noticeably later than others'.
Fine-Motor Planning: Hands	☐ May have difficulty with manual tasks, including drawing, writing, buttoning, opening snack packages, using eating utensils, doing jigsaw puzzles, playing with and cleaning up Legos.
Fine-Motor Planning: Eyes	☐ May have difficulty using both eyes together, tracking moving objects, focusing, and shifting gaze from far to near point. May have a problem copying from the blackboard, keeping his place in a book, and organizing desk space. May have sloppy handwriting and poor eye-hand coordination when drawing, creating art projects, building with blocks, or tying shoes.
Fine-Motor Planning: Mouth	☐ May have difficulty sucking on a nipple or through a straw; eating, chewing, and swallowing; blowing bubbles and breathing; holding mouth closed. May drool excessively. May have problem articulating speech sounds and speaking clearly enough to be understood (by age of three).

WHAT SPD IS NOT:
"LOOK-ALIKE" SYMPTOMS

Many symptoms of SPD look like symptoms of other common disabilities. Indeed, so many symptoms overlap that differentiating one difficulty from another may be difficult. For example, if a child is inattentive and often has difficulty staying focused on tasks or play activities, he may have SPD. Similarly, if the child is hyperactive, often fidgeting or squirming, he may have SPD.

But—might something else be going on? Yes, indeed. An alternative diagnosis may be that the child has Attention-Deficit/Hyperactivity Disorder (ADHD), learning disabilities (LD), poor auditory or visual discrimination, speech/language problems, allergies, nutritional deficiencies, an emotional problem—or that he is behaving just like a typical child!

Some children have only SPD. Others have SPD in addition to one or more other disabilities, such as ADHD and LD. The overlapping circles in the diagram on page 22 illustrate the relationship of these three common problems that can affect children's behavior. Please understand that ADHD and LD are just two of the many disorders, including autism, with which SPD can overlap.

So, how can one tell the difference between SPD and other disabilities? *The red flags are a child's unusual responses to touching and being touched or to moving and being moved.*

The descriptions below provide information about some of the other problems associated with SPD.

ASSOCIATED PROBLEMS

A democratic disorder, SPD affects people of all ages, races, and cognitive skills, all over the world. Diverse populations include those with severe neurological disabilities, mild cerebral palsy and autism spectrum disorders, premature babies, sensory-deprived children in Eastern European orphanages, and highly gifted children. Although

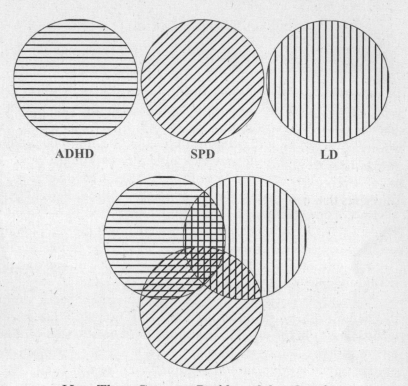

ADHD **SPD** **LD**

How Three Common Problems May Overlap

these children may not seem to have much in common, they frequently experience similar problems in processing sensations.

Although SPD can stand alone, it often coexists with—and complicates—other problems. For instance, if a child has autism, he may also have overresponsivity to touch. The sensory problem does not cause autism, but it certainly exacerbates it. The more difficulty a child has in one area, the more difficulty he is likely to have in others. This is especially true with neurological disabilities, which are on a continuum.

Please be aware that the problems discussed below may have a sensory processing component—or they may be caused by another developmental problem altogether.

Regulatory Disorders

SELF-REGULATION

The child may have difficulty modulating (adjusting) his mood. He may be unable to "rev up," or to calm down once aroused. He may become fussy easily. He may have difficulty with self-comforting after being hurt or upset. Delaying gratification and tolerating transitions from one activity to another may be hard. The child may perform unevenly: "with it" one day, "out of it" the next. Therapy, a "sensory diet" and nutritional supplements are some of the treatments that may help (see Chapter Nine).

SLEEPING

Falling asleep, staying asleep, and waking up may be problematic. The child with SPD may need an unusually long afternoon nap, or she may never nap even if exhausted. Because a sleep disorder is often caused by a separation problem, she may want to sleep with her parents. She may have trouble comforting herself to sleep, or may constantly awaken during the night.

Sleep problems may be associated with a high need for movement. If the child has not had her quota of movement during the day, her arousal levels may fluctuate erratically, and she may become overaroused at night.

Over- or underresponsivity also may cause the child to feel uncomfortable in bed. The pajamas or sheets may feel scratchy. The pillowcase may not smell right, especially after its familiar, ripe scent has been washed out. The blankets may be too heavy or not heavy enough.

Sensory integration treatment addresses the underlying problem, which is poor regulation of arousal and self-calming. Until this issue is "put to rest," try these suggestions to help a child fall and stay asleep:

- During the day—plenty of movement, such as swinging and jogging; hard work, such as carrying laundry baskets; dietary supplements that calm the brain, such as magnesium, essential fatty acids, and GABA (gamma-aminobutyric acid); no foods with additives including aspartame, MSG and artificial colors, which excite the brain

• Before going to bed—a warm bath and then right into bed; no TV or computer time for a couple of hours before bed

• In bed—one great story; a back massage and deep joint compression to the shoulders, arms and legs; a tight tuck-in under a weighted blanket; and saying, "Just *pretend* to sleep"

• After the tuck-in—a night light if the child is afraid of the dark; sleepy sounds, e.g., Bach or Mozart adagios; Genevieve Jereb's *Cool Bananas*, or white noise such as the sound of rain or waves; and your own parental resolve!

EATING

Settling down to eat may be a challenge for the out-of-sync child. One reason may be overresponsivity to tactile sensations. The texture and consistency of the mashed potatoes, rice pudding, applesauce, or turkey burger may be intolerable in a sensitive mouth. Tactile oversensitivity in the mouth is also called "oral defensiveness."

Another reason may be that the food looks, smells, or tastes yucky. A picky eater may have trouble getting the food to his mouth because of inefficient processing of sensations coming from the muscles (proprioception). Or he may need to concentrate not on eating but on staying seated because of inefficient processing about where he is in space and whether he is sitting up or falling off his chair (the vestibular system).

Still another reason may be that the child has not developed a basic sensory-motor pattern involving the coordination of sucking, swallowing, and breathing. The result is poor oral-motor skills, which affect chewing and eating solid food, trying new food, keeping food down, digesting food, and so forth.

Whatever the reason for selective eating, the picky eater has unusual food preferences or a limited food repertoire. He may eat only crispy foods, such as bacon and crackers, or only soft foods, such as yogurt and macaroni and cheese, or only cold or hot foods. He may crave sour foods, such as pickles, and sweets, such as sugary snacks and juice. As a result, nutritional deficits and cravings may affect his development, weight, and stamina and cause him to have behavioral ups and downs, much like a yo-yo.

Usually absent from the picky eater's diet, and thus from his body and brain, are essential fatty acids, B vitamins, minerals, and fat-soluble antioxidants. A child who rejects peanut butter, broccoli, spinach, beans, and sweet potatoes, for example, may get insufficient magnesium, an essential mineral. A magnesium deficiency may lead to hearing damage, auditory processing problems, muscle spasms, restless sleep, and sensory-motor difficulties associated with frequent ear infections. A deficiency in zinc (found in eggs, peanuts, bran, cocoa, etc.) may affect the child's sense of taste and, thus, her interest in food. It may also lead to low muscle tone, auditory and visual problems, rashes and "fly away" hair.

Here are some suggestions to improve your child's eating:

- Get rid of junk food

- Provide nutritional supplements, especially Omega-3 fats (found in flaxseeds, walnuts, and salmon), because the nervous system is made up of about 60 percent fat

- Provide a vibrating toothbrush or facial/oral massager to desensitize the child's lips and mouth

- Take the child for sensory integration and provide a sensory diet at home. (See Chapter Nine.)

DIGESTION AND ELIMINATION

What goes in comes out. What doesn't go in doesn't come out. The picky eater who pushes away nourishing foods with naturally bright color, varied texture and lots of fiber—the stuff of stool, if you will—is likely to have chronic diarrhea or constipation.

Aside from the sensory-based problem of picky eating, SPD may affect digestion and elimination in other ways. The child may not recognize signals of thirst, hunger, and satiety (fullness). This poor awareness of internal organs is a problem with interoception, which is sensitivity to stimuli coming from inside the body. Another cause of poor digestion is inactivity. The child who is sedentary because of difficulty moving his body may also have difficulty moving his bowels.

Tactile problems may contribute to toileting issues. Under-responsivity to tactile sensations may mean that the child does not perceive wetness, and so he may not develop efficient bladder control. (Thick disposable diapers that carry wetness away to keep the child comfortably dry are part of the problem!) He may develop enuresis (en-yu-ree-sis) and become a chronic bed-wetter.

Or, if he is a sensory seeker, he may actually *like* how a fully loaded diaper or pair of underpants feels. Or smells.

In addition, inefficient proprioception (the "body position sense," or the "muscle sense," discussed in Chapter Five) may affect the child's muscle tone and make it hard for him to "hold it." A problem with postural control may make it difficult to stay poised on the toilet seat. A problem with the vestibular sense may make him feel unbalanced and ungrounded, as if he is falling off the toilet—or worse, in.

Suggestions include:

• Plenty of water, fiber, and active movement throughout the day

• Telephone book, box, or stool under the child's feet to help him feel grounded

• Working with an occupational therapist, nutritionist, or other professional with expertise in eating disorders and sensory processing

AROUSAL, ACTIVITY LEVEL, AND ATTENTION
Arousal, activity level, and attention are self-regulation problems that frequently coexist with SPD.

• Unusually high arousal and activity level: The child may be always on the go, restless, and fidgety. He may move with short and nervous gestures, play or work aimlessly, be quick-tempered and excitable, and find it impossible to stay seated.

• Unusually low arousal and activity level: The child may move slowly and in a daze, fatigue easily, lack initiative and "stick-to-it-tiveness," and show little interest in the world. She may have been an easy baby—in fact, a *too* easy baby, who nestled into anybody's arms, rarely complained, slept more than other children, and needed to be fed and dressed later than others.

• Inattention: Perhaps because of sensory over- or under-responsiveness, the child may have a short attention span, even for activities he enjoys. He may be highly distractible, paying attention to everything except the task at hand. He may be disorganized and forgetful.

• Impulsivity: To get or avoid sensory stimulation, the child may be heedlessly energetic and impetuous. She may lack self-control and be unable to stop after starting an activity. She may pour juice until it spills, run pell-mell into people, overturn toy bins, and talk out of turn.

SOCIAL AND EMOTIONAL FUNCTIONING
Another coexisting regulatory problem may be how the child feels about himself and relates to other people.

• Poor adaptability: The child may resist meeting new people, trying new games or toys or tasting different foods. He may have difficulty making transitions from one situation to another. The child may seem stubborn and uncooperative when it is time to leave the house, come for dinner, get into or out of the bathtub, or change from a reading to a math activity. Minor changes in routine will readily upset this child who does not "go with the flow."

• Attachment problem: The child may have separation anxiety and be clingy and fearful when apart from one or two "significant olders." Or, she may physically avoid her parents, teachers, and others in her circle.

• Frustration: Struggling to accomplish tasks that peers do easily, the child may give up quickly. He may be a perfectionist and become upset when art projects, dramatic play, or homework assignments are not going as well as he expects.

• Difficulty with friendships: The child may be hard to get along with and have problems making and keeping friends. Insisting on dictating all the rules and being the winner, the best, or the first, he may be a poor game-player. He may need to control his surrounding territory, be in the "driver's seat," and have trouble sharing toys.

• Poor communication: The child may have difficulty verbally in the way she articulates her speech, "gets the words out," and writes. She may have difficulty expressing her thoughts, feelings, and needs, not only through words but also nonverbally through gestures, body language, and facial expressions.

• Other emotional problems: He may be inflexible, irrational, and overly sensitive to change, stress, and hurt feelings. Demanding and needy, he may seek attention in negative ways. He may be angry or panicky for no obvious reason. He may be unhappy, believing and saying that he is dumb, crazy, no good, a loser, and a failure. *Low self-esteem is one of the most telling symptoms of Sensory Processing Disorder.*

• Academic problems: The child may have difficulty learning new skills and concepts. Although bright, the child may be perceived as an underachiever.

Please note: Many children with SPD have behavior problems. However, most children with behavior problems do not have SPD! Every child is occasionally out-of-sync. Careful diagnosis is imperative to determine which symptoms are related to sensory processing problems, and which are not.

Attention-Deficit/Hyperactivity Disorder (ADHD)

While SPD is not the same as its "look-alike" ADHD, the two disorders may simultaneously affect the out-of-sync child. Attention-Deficit/Hyperactivity Disorder (ADHD) is an umbrella term for a problem interfering with one's ability to attend to and stay focused on meaningful tasks, control his impulses, and regulate his activity level. Symptoms of this neurologically based disorder are hyperactivity, inattention (distractibility) and/or impulsivity.

Determining if the child has one and not the other matters, because treatments for the two problems differ. Treatment for ADHD often involves behavior management and other psychological approaches, as well as psychostimulants such as Ritalin, to make the child's brain available for learning.

Dr. Lucy Jane Miller, PhD, is the principle investigator in the field of sensory processing research at The Children's Hospital of Denver. She collaborates with other occupational therapists to define the underlying neurological and physiological foundations of SPD. The goals of this rigorous research include: 1) distinguishing SPD from ADHD and other disabilities, and 2) determining the best treatment for children with different types of SPD, because one treatment does not fit all.

Among the researchers' findings is evidence that many children with SPD differ from children with ADHD in their responses to unexpected sensations, such as light touches, loud noises, flickering lights, strong smells, and being tilted backward in a chair. Children with ADHD tend to alert to these novel sensations and then, like most people, habituate—i.e., become easily accustomed—to them. Life goes on.

Some children with SPD, however, may not alert to these everyday sensations. Life does not affect them much. Other children with SPD may be continually on alert and may not become accustomed to the sensations at all. Life affects them too much.

Outside the research laboratory, parents and teachers may notice other differences between SPD and ADHD. For instance, many children with SPD prefer the "same-old, same-old" in a familiar and predictable environment, while children with ADHD prefer novelty and diversion. Many children with SPD have poor motor coordination, while children with ADHD often shine in sports. Many children with SPD have adequate impulse control, unless bothered by sensations, while children with ADHD often have poor impulse control.

Another difference is that medicine may help the child with ADHD, but medicine will not solve the problem of SPD. Therapy focusing on sensory integration and a sensory diet of purposeful activities help the child with SPD.

Learning Disability

A learning disability (LD) can be defined in many ways.

1) Simple definition: A learning disability is difficulty in the Four R's—Reading, 'Riting, 'Rithmetic, and Relationships.

2) Clinical definition: A learning disability is a neurological problem in processing information that causes difficulties mastering academic skills and strategies. A breakdown occurs in one of the four steps involved in learning: input (taking in information from the senses), integration (processing and interpreting the information), memory (using, storing, and retrieving the information), and output (sending out the information through language or motor activities).

3) Formal definition: Our federal law, *Individuals with Disabilities Education Improvement Act of 2004 (IDEA 04)*, defines a specific learning disability as "a disorder in one or more of the basic psychological processes involved in understanding or in using language, spoken or written, that may manifest itself in an imperfect ability to listen, think, speak, read, write, spell, or to do mathematical calculations."

While SPD may affect the child's auditory, visual, and motor skills and her ability to process and sequence information, it is not, at present, specifically identified as an eligible, qualifying disability. Thus, it does not necessarily make a child eligible for special education and related services, such as occupational, physical, or speech/language therapy. A child with SPD may be eligible for services if SPD coexists with an eligible disability and contributes to a child's difficulties with participation in her educational program.

Dyslexia

Dyslexia is a common difficulty in reading, writing and spelling, despite a person's intelligence and motivation. Dyslexia is many things: a neurological disorder; a hereditary, familial problem; a specific learning disability; and a syndrome, i.e., a group of related characteristics varying in severity from one individual to another.

Sensations of sight, sound, and movement are involved in reading. The problem is in the way different brain parts simultaneously process the sensory components of reading. The timing involved in analyzing a word is out of sync, preventing instantaneous, automatic word recognition.

Children with this multisensory syndrome can benefit from multisensory intervention, integrating visual, aural, tactile and kinesthetic (i.e., sight, sound, touch and movement) experiences.

Autism

Autism is a neurobiological disorder. The structures of the brains of people with autism are atypical. Research is pointing to differences in overall brain size and the numbers of certain cells; to abnormalities in the cerebellum that affect motor, sensory, language, cognitive and attention functions; and to altered genes that interfere with brain development. A new "underconnectivity theory" suggests that autism interferes with efficient integration, timing, and synchronization of brain activation patterns.

Autism, or the umbrella term, Autistic Spectrum Disorders (ASD), is not one thing but many. Like SPD and LD, the term autism encompasses a wide array of symptoms. In broad terms, autism is a Pervasive Developmental Disorder (PDD) that affects verbal and nonverbal communication, social interaction, imagination, and problem-solving. Autism is usually evident before the child turns three and greatly affects educational performance. It causes the child to engage in repetitive motions and have a narrow repertoire of activities and interests.

Another component of autism—and a very important one—is difficulty with sensory modulation, sensory discrimination, motor planning, and sequencing. Problems with sensations are sometimes overlooked or downplayed but are among the main areas of impairment.

Every child with autism has a unique pattern of these challenges. For example, one autistic child may have excellent visual discrimination and be an incredibly talented artist but have poor auditory discrimination and relatively little language. Another child may have excellent auditory skills and remember song lyrics, compose rhymes, and enjoy stories, but have poor visual discrimination and meager motor-planning skills.

Most children with autism have poor regulation, or modulation, of ordinary sensations. For some, the capacity to regulate touch, movement, sound, and visual stimuli will always be troublesome. However, for others, environmental sensitivity can be a bonus. For example, a keen sensitivity to sounds, including perfect pitch, may lead to a career in music.

A spokesperson for autism, Temple Grandin, PhD, eloquently describes the torment of sensory stimulation. As a child, being touched and hugged by another person made her feel like a wild animal, until she designed a squeeze machine—her "hug box"—to satisfy her craving for the sensation of being held. Hearing ordinary sounds still makes her heart race and her ears hurt, unless she "shuts off " her ears by engaging in rhythmic, stereotypical autistic behavior.

Whereas little Temple avoided touch and sound sensations, she craved visual sensations. "I loved striped shirts and Day-Glo paint," she writes, "and I loved to watch supermarket sliding doors go back and forth." Equipped with intense visualization skills, and simpatico with animals, Dr. Grandin grew up to earn her doctorate in animal science. Today, she specializes in the design of humane livestock-handling facilities.

That most people with autism have some degree of SPD is a recognized fact. Understanding how sensory and motor problems complicate the child's daily life is crucial for designing an appropriate intervention program. Parents must ensure that their child's treatment program includes ample sensory-motor experiences and an individualized sensory diet. (See Chapter Nine.)

Asperger Syndrome

A subtype of autism and another form of PDD is Asperger Syndrome (AS). Most characteristics are similar to those of autism. Exceptions are that the child with AS may function better in social situations and at school and that he uses more typical speech and thinking patterns. Often the child is dubbed a "Little Professor," because of his extraordinary depth of knowledge about a particular subject, such as the Civil War, railroads, the planetary system, and so forth.

People with Asperger Syndrome tend to be anxious, poorly coordinated, and eccentric. They frequently have difficulties with hearing, vision, moving, touching, and other sensory areas. Sensory integration treatment often will lessen their anxiety and clumsiness and improve their social participation.

Nonverbal Learning Disorder

Nonverbal Learning Disorder (NLD) is a neurological syndrome that causes a person to have difficulty interpreting and understanding nonverbal cues in the environment. The name of the disorder may be confusing, because it seems to imply that the person is nonverbal. In fact, the person is quite verbal and expresses himself well; it is the nonverbal parts of communication like smiles and waves that he has trouble interpreting.

One of the major deficits of the child is difficulty processing sensory information. SPD underlies the child's problems with coordination and balance, visual discrimination, and the ability to comprehend gestures, facial expressions, and social cues. For children with NLD, sensory integration therapy can be very beneficial.

Psychological Problems

SPD is a physical problem, not a psychological problem, per se. It may certainly overlap with, and add to, psychological problems. As the child matures, serious psychological problems may develop, indeed, if the underlying SPD is neither recognized nor addressed early. The inability to cope with emotional, physical, and social challenges is often present by the age of three or four if sensory integration intervention has not yet begun.

Distinguishing SPD from mental and emotional disorders is as important as distinguishing it from ADHD, because the treatments vary greatly. Unfortunately, symptoms of SPD are often misinterpreted as psychological problems.

An example is Obsessive-Compulsive Disorder (OCD). Say a child washes her hands many times a day. Repetitive hand washing is a common symptom of OCD. But is it possible that the child goes frequently to the sink to wash away tactile sensations from her oversensitive palms?

Another look-alike problem is Bipolar Disorder. A child with this psychological disability shows many symptoms that a child with SPD may have: depression or sadness, difficulty falling asleep, risk-taking behavior, extreme sensitivity to sensory stimuli, difficulty engaging in play, reluctance to engage in novel tasks, fidgetiness, and so forth. Could the problem be manic depression—could it be SPD—or could it be both?

Selective Mutism

Selective Mutism (SM) is a childhood anxiety disorder. It is characterized by a child's inability to speak and communicate comfortably in select social settings, such as school or a friend's house, where answering questions and having conversations are expected. A child with Selective Mutism is able to talk normally in settings where she feels secure and relaxed, such as home.

In addition to this debilitating social anxiety, children with SM often have SPD. They may withdraw from some sensations and seek others, such as playground swinging.

Experts speculate that sensory processing problems play a role in triggering the overwhelming anxiety that causes some children to withdraw and become mute. Addressing sensory needs is a successful means to help them "get the words out."

Genetic Syndromes

A host of other disorders and genetic syndromes are characterized by sensory problems.

Down Syndrome is a congenital disorder caused by an extra chromosome. The condition alters the typical development of the brain and body, causes mental retardation and affects the child's sensory processing. Common problems include poor muscle tone and difficulties with fine-motor and gross-motor skills that affect movement and coordination, play and self-care, speech and eating.

Fragile X Syndrome, a congenital disorder, is caused by a mutation in a gene that makes up the X chromosome. More boys than girls are affected. Sensory processing issues may include over- or underresponsivity to sensations, such as touch, movement and sounds; sensory-based motor difficulties, affecting body awareness, motor planning and coordination; and problems with sustaining attention and regulating arousal level.

Fetal Alcohol Syndrome (FAS), or Fetal Alcohol Effects (FAE), is a nongenetic disability: it is noninherited and is preventable. It affects the baby whose mother drinks alcohol during pregnancy. The child may be small and have physical abnormalities of the face, bones, and organs. He may have difficulty taking in sensory information, processing it and making adaptive responses, especially in social situations. He may withdraw from touches and sounds, simultaneously seeking movement. Sensory issues may lead to speech and language delays, emotional instability, hyperactivity, and learning disabilities.

Syndromes that coexist with SPD—and often go misdiagnosed—include Angelman, CHARGE, Dandy-Walker, Ehlers-Danlos, Prader-Willi, Russell-Silver, Smith-Lemli-Opitz, and Williams. For children with these syndromes, occupational therapy using a sensory integration framework can improve motor, social, and language skills. Other therapies, including physical therapy and speech/language therapy, may help as well, especially when they include sensory integration.

Allergies

SPD often coexists with allergies. The child may suffer from allergic reactions to dust, pollens, molds, grass, fur, and, of course, foods. The casein in dairy products and the gluten in wheat are the big culprits. Additionally, the chemicals in food, medicines, and the air we inhale may be toxic for the child with a sensitive system. These allergens can harm his developing nervous system, causing learning and behavior problems.

In her classic books, Doris Rapp, MD, discusses the predominant symptoms of allergies, including the allergic nose rub ("allergic salute"), red circles under the eyes ("allergic shiners"), irritability, depression, aggression, and under- or overresponsiveness to sensory stimulation, particularly sound and touch.

Medicine is not the antidote. The solution for many children is identifying and eliminating irritating foods, such as milk or wheat, and environmental irritants, such as stuffed animals and mold. Try it—and watch how many symptoms associated with allergies and sensory processing disorders clear up dramatically, and without side effects.

POSSIBLE CAUSES OF SPD

The problems discussed above may coexist with SPD but do not cause it. The cause may be one of these factors:

1) A genetic or hereditary predisposition, often the case if the child's parent, sibling, or other close relative has some SPD

2) Prenatal circumstances, including:

- chemicals, medications or toxins like lead poisoning that the fetus absorbs

- the mother's smoking or drug or alcohol abuse

- unpreventable pregnancy complications, such as a virus, a chronic illness, great emotional stress or a problem with the placenta

- multiple births (e.g., twins or triplets)

3) Prematurity or low birth weight

4) Birth trauma, perhaps due to an emergency cesarean section, a lack of oxygen, or surgery soon after birth

5) Postnatal circumstances, including:

- environmental pollutants

- excessive stimulation, such as child abuse or warfare

- insufficient stimulation and limited opportunities to move, play, and interact with others

- lengthy hospitalization

- institutionalization in an orphanage, such as in Romania or another Eastern European country

6) Unknown reasons

Exciting research is answering many questions about the disorder. Dr. Ayres' explorations, decades ago, laid the foundation for current research, such as sophisticated quantitative or functional brain imaging studies that demonstrate anatomical differences in the brains of out-of-sync children. As researchers make clearer distinctions among those with sensory issues, increased knowledge about the roots of SPD will lead to the most effective interventions.

WHO HAS SENSORY PROCESSING DISORDER?

On a bell-shaped curve of humanity, some people have a poorly integrated neurological system, some have an excellent one, and the rest of us fall somewhere in the middle.

Think about people who are graceful and popular, like ballerinas, athletes, charismatic politicians, and delightful children. These people may be blessed with exceptionally efficient sensory processing.

Now, think about people you know who have problems functioning in certain aspects of their lives. They may be clumsy, have few friends, or show neither common sense nor self-control. They may have SPD.

SPD is on a continuum, says nutritionist Kelly Dorfman. At one end of the continuum, some people have mild dysfunction that affects their self-regulation.

At the far end of the continuum, many people with autism have severe sensory processing issues, further complicating their profound difficulties with learning, communication, and relationships. Along the SI continuum are those with ADHD, Asperger syndrome and other pervasive developmental delays.

We know that SPD intensifies the bigger problems of children with the disorders, syndromes and environmental conditions mentioned above. For all these children, remediation of their sensory issues through occupational therapy has an overall, positive effect.

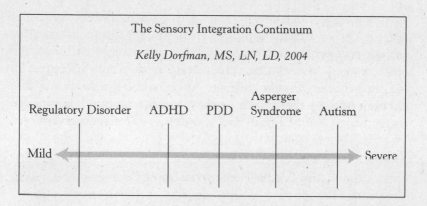

The Sensory Integration Continuum

Kelly Dorfman, MS, LN, LD, 2004

| Regulatory Disorder | ADHD | PDD | Asperger Syndrome | Autism |

Mild ⟵————————————————⟶ Severe

We also know that some "normal" children, who are not regarded as having any significant or diagnosable problems, have SPD. These children, whom intervention also helps, are the focus of this book.

What percentage of "normal" children is challenged by inefficient sensory processing? Statistics are slippery and depend on the criteria used. In 1979, Dr. Ayres estimated that 5 percent to 10 percent of children have sensory processing problems significant enough to warrant intervention. In 2004, a study to determine the prevalence of SPD provided a similarly conservative estimate. Based on my anecdotal observations as a teacher, I guesstimate that the numbers are higher—more like 10 percent to 15 percent.

Occupational therapists commonly note that approximately 80 percent of these children are boys, but this statistic is open to dispute. Many professionals believe that girls are just as likely as boys to have neurological disorders, including SPD, ADHD, and learning disabilities. Girls, however, frequently do not display the same behavior problems that attract attention, so they tend to go unnoticed—and to fall through the cracks.

Should we be alarmed by the increasing numbers of children identified as having SPD? Are we indiscriminately sticking labels on children? Are we just "looking for something wrong"?

No, no, no!

In fact, identifying children with SPD is a positive step. As we learn more about the mechanics of the human brain, we are finally understanding why some children are out of sync. And now—we can do something to help!

DON'T WE ALL EXPERIENCE SOME SENSORY PROCESSING PROBLEMS?

From time to time, we all experience some problems processing sensations. Too much or too little sensory stimulation confuses the brain and can cause temporary discomfort. Illness, fatigue, and stress can also interfere with smooth functioning.

For example, attending a noisy, crowded party can be overwhelming. Taking a bumpy airplane ride can overload your brain with rapid movement sensations. Lingering in bed with the flu can prevent you from receiving sufficient movement experiences and make you feel weak. Walking from a well-lit room into a dark closet can deprive your eyes of light and therefore your brain of visual sensations.

Not being in control of oneself is very unpleasant, but an occasional disorganizing experience is normal. It is when the brain is so disorganized that a person has difficulty functioning in daily life that the person is diagnosed as having Sensory Processing Disorder.

SAMPLE SENSORY-MOTOR HISTORY QUESTIONNAIRE

Below is a sample questionnaire similar to those that parents or teachers complete when a child begins to be evaluated by an occupational therapist. A questionnaire helps the therapist learn about the child's sensory-motor history. After analyzing it, the therapist determines whether the child needs treatment and, if so, uses it to design an individualized program, or sensory diet (see Chapter Nine).

This questionnaire was designed by Sharon Cermak and Alice Miller at Sargent College, Boston University, in the 1990s. It is applicable to all children today, although its original purpose was to examine the sensory processing characteristics of children who have been adopted from Eastern European countries. The questionnaire is based on the work of Winnie Dunn, PhD, and the therapists at Occupational Therapy Associates-Watertown, PC, and is abbreviated here with their gracious permission.

Take some time to study the questions. They will help you understand how sensory processing affects your child's overall development. Some questions pertain to the child's responses to sensations, including touch, movement, vision, hearing, taste, and smell. Other questions pertain to the child's self-regulation and behavior, including activity level, feeding, organization and attention, sleeping, and social-emotional skills, all of which are strongly influenced by sensory processing.

Before picking up your pencil, you may want to make a few clean copies of the questionnaire to share with your child's teacher, caregiver, or grandparent. (Most of the questions are applicable to preschoolers and elementary age children.) Many checks under the "Often" column suggest that SPD affects your child and that a professional diagnosis is in order.

SENSORY-MOTOR HISTORY QUESTIONNAIRE FOR PARENTS OF YOUNG CHILDREN

Prepared by Sharon Cermak, EdD, OTR, et al.

SENSES

I. *Touch:* Does your child . . .

    1. Avoid or dislike getting hands messy?

                    Often_____ Sometimes_____ Rarely_____

2. Become upset when face is washed?

Often_____ Sometimes_____ Rarely_____

3. Become upset when having hair combed or fingernails cut?

Often_____ Sometimes_____ Rarely_____

4. Prefer long-sleeved clothing or jackets, even when it is hot?

Often_____ Sometimes_____ Rarely_____

5. Avoid wearing clothes made of certain fabrics?

Often_____ Sometimes_____ Rarely_____

6. Have trouble changing clothing when seasons change?

Often_____ Sometimes_____ Rarely_____

7. Avoid going barefoot, especially in sand or grass?

Often_____ Sometimes_____ Rarely_____

8. Become irritated by tags on clothing?

Often_____ Sometimes_____ Rarely_____

9. Complain if socks are not on correctly?

Often_____ Sometimes_____ Rarely_____

10. Complain about bumps on bed sheets?

Often_____ Sometimes_____ Rarely_____

11. Seem to crave being held or cuddled?

Often_____ Sometimes_____ Rarely_____

12. Express discomfort when touched in a friendly way by others? Often_____ Sometimes_____ Rarely_____

13. Prefer to touch others rather than be touched by them?

Often_____ Sometimes_____ Rarely_____

14. Tend to bump or push others?

Often_____ Sometimes_____ Rarely_____

15. Seem excessively ticklish?

Often_____ Sometimes_____ Rarely_____

16. Seem overly-sensitive to pain, and be bothered by small cuts? Often_____ Sometimes_____ Rarely_____

17. Show an unusual need to touch certain textures, surfaces, toys? Often_____ Sometimes_____ Rarely_____

18. Mouth objects or clothing often?

        Often____ Sometimes____ Rarely____

19. Have difficulty judging how much strength to use, e.g., petting animals with too much force?

        Often____ Sometimes____ Rarely____

II. *Movement*: Does your child . . .

1. Become anxious or distressed when feet leave the ground?

        Often____ Sometimes____ Rarely____

2. Avoid climbing or jumping?

        Often____ Sometimes____ Rarely____

3. Appear reluctant to participate in sports and motor games?

        Often____ Sometimes____ Rarely____

4. Seem fearful of catching balls?

        Often____ Sometimes____ Rarely____

5. Show fear of falling or heights?

        Often____ Sometimes____ Rarely____

6. Dislike elevators or escalators?

        Often____ Sometimes____ Rarely____

7. Dislike riding in a car?

        Often____ Sometimes____ Rarely____

8. Dislike activities where head is upside down (as with hair washing) or when lifted overhead (as in somersaults)?

        Often____ Sometimes____ Rarely____

9. Love to be tipped upside down or lifted overhead?

        Often____ Sometimes____ Rarely____

10. Seek out all kinds of movement activities?

        Often____ Sometimes____ Rarely____

11. Enjoy merry-go-rounds and fast rides?

        Often____ Sometimes____ Rarely____

12. Jump often and for long time on beds or other bouncy surfaces?

        Often____ Sometimes____ Rarely____

13. Like to spin himself/herself ?

        Often_____ Sometimes_____ Rarely_____

14. Rock his/her body or head?

        Often_____ Sometimes_____ Rarely_____

15. Bang head on purpose?

        Often_____ Sometimes_____ Rarely_____

16. Throw him/herself against floor, wall, or other people for fun?   Often_____ Sometimes_____ Rarely_____

17. Take unusual risks during play?

        Often_____ Sometimes_____ Rarely_____

III. *Visual*: Does your child . . .

1. Become easily distracted by visual stimulation?

        Often_____ Sometimes_____ Rarely_____

2. Express discomfort at bright lights?

        Often_____ Sometimes_____ Rarely_____

3. Avoid or have difficulty with direct eye contact?

        Often_____ Sometimes_____ Rarely_____

4. Have a hard time picking out a single object from many, such as finding a specific toy in a toy box?

        Often_____ Sometimes_____ Rarely_____

IV. *Auditory*: Does your child . . .

1. Become distracted or have a problem when surrounded by a lot of noise?   Often_____ Sometimes_____ Rarely_____

2. Respond negatively to unexpected or loud noises?

        Often_____ Sometimes_____ Rarely_____

3. Like to make loud noises?

        Often_____ Sometimes_____ Rarely_____

V. *Taste and Smell*: Does your child . . .

    1. Explore objects by smelling them?
                Often____ Sometimes____ Rarely____

    2. Seem bothered by smells that most other people do not notice?   Often____ Sometimes____ Rarely____

    3. Chew or lick nonfood items?
                Often____ Sometimes____ Rarely____

SENSORY-RELATED SKILLS

I. *Activity Level*: Does your child . . .

    1. Tend to be especially active and always on the go?
                Often____ Sometimes____ Rarely____

    2. Tend to fidget excessively in a chair when eating or working?
                Often____ Sometimes____ Rarely____

    3. Tend to lack carefulness and to be impulsive?
                Often____ Sometimes____ Rarely____

    4. Seem aggressive in play?
                Often____ Sometimes____ Rarely____

II. *Feeding*: Does your child . . .

    1. Need assistance to feed himself/herself?
                Often____ Sometimes____ Rarely____

    2. Tend to eat in a sloppy manner?
                Often____ Sometimes____ Rarely____

    3. Frequently spill liquids?
                Often____ Sometimes____ Rarely____

    4. Drool?   Often____ Sometimes____ Rarely____

    5. Have trouble chewing?
                Often____ Sometimes____ Rarely____

6. Have trouble swallowing?

        Often____ Sometimes____ Rarely____

7. Have difficulty or dislike eating foods with lumps, such as chunky soups?   Often____ Sometimes____ Rarely____

8. Stuff or put too much food in his/her mouth at once?

        Often____ Sometimes____ Rarely____

III. *Organization*: Does your child . . .

1. Frequently lose things, such as homework or coat?

        Often____ Sometimes____ Rarely____

2. Get lost easily?   Often____ Sometimes____ Rarely____

3. Have difficulty tolerating changes in plans or expectations?

        Often____ Sometimes____ Rarely____

4. Have difficulty changing from one activity to another?

        Often____ Sometimes____ Rarely____

5. Need extra assistance to get started with a task or activity?

        Often____ Sometimes____ Rarely____

6. Become easily distracted while working or playing?

        Often____ Sometimes____ Rarely____

7. Have a short attention span?

        Often____ Sometimes____ Rarely____

IV. *Sleeping*: Does your child . . .

1. Have irregular sleep patterns?

        Often____ Sometimes____ Rarely____

2. Wake frequently during the night?

        Often____ Sometimes____ Rarely____

3. Have a difficult time falling asleep?

        Often____ Sometimes____ Rarely____

4. Require less sleep than other children?

        Often____ Sometimes____ Rarely____

V. *Social-emotional*: Does your child . . .

1. Have trouble getting along with other children his/her age?

    Often_____ Sometimes_____ Rarely_____

2. Seem overly sensitive to criticism?

    Often_____ Sometimes_____ Rarely_____

3. Seem overly anxious or fearful?

    Often_____ Sometimes _____ Rarely_____

4. Tend to be quiet or withdrawn?

    Often_____ Sometimes_____ Rarely_____

5. Tend to be easily frustrated?

    Often_____ Sometimes_____ Rarely_____

6. Tend to be unusually uncooperative or stubborn?

    Often_____ Sometimes_____ Rarely_____

7. Have temper tantrums or outbursts of anger?

    Often_____ Sometimes_____ Rarely_____

8. Seem to need more protection from life than other children?

    Often_____ Sometimes_____ Rarely_____

HOPE IS AT HAND

Having looked at the questionnaire, you should be getting a feel for how SPD can get in a child's way. If you (and the teacher) checked "Often" many times, you may believe you have an out-of-sync child. You may be asking: Is my child's development out of my hands? Will my child become an out-of-sync adult?

Not necessarily. Your child may develop into a self-regulating, functioning grown-up if he or she receives understanding, support, and early intervention.

Early intervention involves treatment designed to correct or prevent the young child's developmental delays or disabilities. Treatment for SPD usually comes in the form of occupational therapy in a sensory integration framework (see Chapter Eight).

With treatment, the child can become as competent as possible—physically, academically, and emotionally.

Young children respond well to early intervention, because their central nervous systems are still flexible, or "plastic." Plasticity means that children's brain functioning is not fixed; it can change or be changed.

As children grow, their brains become less malleable and their unusual reactions to sensations become more established. If your child is older than a preschooler, however, don't give up hope! Older children and even adults benefit from therapy, too. It is never too late to get help.

For the child with severe sensory dysfunction, treatment is crucial. For the child with moderate or even mild dysfunction, treatment can make a wonderful difference.

How Does Treatment Help?

Treatment helps the child process all the senses, so they can work together. When the child *actively* engages in meaningful activities that provide the intensity, duration, and quality of sensation his central nervous system craves, his adaptive behavior improves. Adaptive behavior leads to better sensory processing. As a result, perceptions, learning, competence, and self-confidence improve. The child becomes able to plan, organize and carry out what he needs and wants to do. Without treatment, SPD may hamper his life in countless ways.

Treatment helps the child now, when he needs assistance to function smoothly. Treatment now helps him build a strong foundation for the future, when life becomes more demanding and complex. Without treatment, SPD persists as a lifelong problem. Indeed, *the child will not grow out of Sensory Processing Disorder, but will grow into it.*

Treatment helps the child develop skills to interact successfully in social situations. The out-of-sync child often lacks the skills to play—and play is every child's primary occupation. Without treatment, SPD interferes with the child's friendships.

Treatment gives the child the tools to become a more efficient learner. Without treatment, SPD interferes with the child's ability to learn, at home, school, and abroad.

Treatment improves the child's emotional well-being. Without treatment, the child who believes she is incompetent may develop into an adult with low self-esteem.

Treatment improves family relationships. As the child responds to sensory challenges with growing self-control, home life becomes more pleasant. With professional support, parents learn to provide consistent discipline and to enjoy their child. In-laws become more empathetic and less critical, and siblings resent the out-of-sync child less. Without treatment, SPD interferes with the interactions and coping skills of everyone in the family.

Johnny is an example of a child who greatly benefited from early intervention. When he was a preschooler, SPD affected his ability to move, play, learn, and relate to others. It affected his posture and balance, hearing and vision, food preferences and sleep patterns. He was fearful, angry, inflexible, and lonely.

Johnny's feet never left the ground because movement made him uncomfortable. He would stand and watch but not join his schoolmates in playground activities. He always carried a stick, as a buffer against the world. When someone approached him, he would brandish the stick and holler, "You're fired!" His sole pleasure was curling up in the quiet corner, peering at a book.

Johnny was one of the first children we screened at St. Columba's Nursery School for SPD. We shared our findings with his parents and suggested occupational therapy, mentioning that early intervention could prevent later problems.

Listening to us, his father folded his arms, scowled, and shook his head. His mother wept and said, "This is all a bad dream."

Although skeptical, his parents decided to take our advice. They took Johnny to a pediatric occupational therapist twice a week. Working with the therapist and his teachers, they devised a sensory diet with activities at home and school to help him become as competent as he could be.

Gradually, Johnny began to participate in some activities. He didn't learn to relish messy play or a rowdy game of tag, but he did learn to paint at the easel and pump on the swing. He stopped carrying his stick in self-defense. He started to use his "indoor" voice instead of bellowing. He found a friend, and then two. He was becoming a real kid.

Today, Johnny is a dream-come-true. Now ten, he plays soccer and basketball. He's a Boy Scout who enjoys camping and climbing rocks. He reads a book every week, for pleasure. Everyone wants to be his friend, because he is reliable and sensitive—in all the right ways. His teacher says, "I wish I had twenty other Johnnys in my classroom."

Johnny's story is true. His dysfunction, once severe, is now mild. He still eats carefully, feels uncomfortable in crowds, avoids escalators, and tends to be a perfectionist. But nobody's perfect!

Not every out-of-sync child will have Johnny's success. Most children do improve, however, when their parents take action. Here are some suggestions:

- Get information and share it with pediatricians, teachers and other caregivers, when appropriate.

- Although difficult to do, accept that the child does not fit your mental image of the perfect child; acknowledge that it is okay and sometimes preferable to have differing abilities.

- Provide the child with a well-balanced sensory diet (Chapter Nine).

- Be patient, consistent and supportive.

- Help the child take control of his or her body and life.

The journey may be long. It may be expensive. It will certainly be frustrating at times. But the journey will also be wonderful and exciting as you learn to help your son or daughter succeed in the occupation of childhood.

Hope is at hand.

Chapter Two

UNDERSTANDING SENSORY
PROCESSING—AND WHAT
CAN GO AMISS

Understanding basic information about sensory processing and Sensory Processing Disorder is important. You need to know about the senses, the developmental stages of sensory processing through which a young child normally progresses, and what happens when sensory processing does not go according to Mother Nature's plan.

THE SENSES

Our senses give us the information we need to function in the world. Their first job is to help us survive. Their second job, after they assure us that we are safe, is to help us learn how to be active, social creatures.

The senses receive information from stimuli both outside and inside our bodies. Every move we make, every bite we eat, every object we touch produces sensations. When we engage in any activity, we use several senses at the same time. The convergence of sensations—especially touch, body position, movement, sight, sound, and smell—is called intersensory integration. This process is key and tells us on the spot what is going on, where, why, and when it matters, and how we must use or respond to it.

The more important the activity, the more senses we use. That is why we use all our senses simultaneously for two very important human activities: eating and procreating.

Sometimes our senses inform us that something in our environment doesn't feel right; we sense that we are in danger and so we respond defensively. For instance, should we feel a tarantula creeping down our neck, we would protect ourselves with a fight-or-flight response. Withdrawing from too much stimulation or from stimulation of the wrong kind is natural.

Sometimes our senses inform us that all is well; we feel safe and satisfied and seek more of the same stimuli. For example, we are so pleased with the taste of one chocolate-covered raisin that we eat a handful.

Sometimes, when we get bored, we go looking for more stimulation. For example, when we have mastered a skill, like ice skating in a straight line, we attempt a more complicated move, like a figure eight.

To do their job well, so that we respond appropriately, the senses must work together. A well-balanced brain that is nourished with many sensations operates well, and when our brain operates smoothly, so do we.

We have more senses than many people realize. Some sensations occur outside our bodies, and some inside.

The External Senses

The sensory systems that receive sensory messages coming from the outside of our body and beyond are sometimes called the external or environmental senses. The information from these senses is called exteroception, referring to the five senses with which we are most familiar:

- The tactile sense, providing information about touch, which we receive through contact with the skin (see Chapter Three),

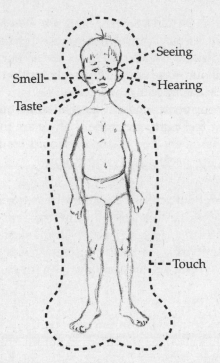

The External (Environmental) Senses

• The olfactory and gustatory senses, providing information about smell and taste, through contact with the nose and mouth, and

• The visual and auditory senses, providing information about sights and sounds coming from "out there" in the environment, without actual contact with our eyes and ears. (See Chapters Six and Seven.) Seeing and hearing are sometimes called the "far senses" because the messages come from a distance.

We are conscious of our external senses, and we have some control over them. We can scrutinize a photograph of the third-grade class to pick out our child's face, or shut our eyes to avoid looking at an unpleasant scene. We can distinguish between a telephone ring and a doorbell, or cover our ears to screen out the dissonance of an untuned violin. We can touch a keyboard letter with one fingertip, or keep our hands jammed in our pockets. As we mature, our brains refine our external senses so that we can respond in a satisfying way to the world around us.

The Internal Senses

When we think about sensory channels, the external senses come first to mind. Less familiar are the internal senses—sometimes called the hidden, special, near, somatosensory ("soma" means "body" in Greek), or body-centered senses. We are unconscious of these senses, yet they are always with us, and we cannot turn them off.

- The interoceptive sense, or interoception, providing information about sensations coming from our internal organs. With a "mind" of its own, it keeps our bodies humming and is essential for survival. It regulates functions such as hunger, thirst, digestion, body temperature, sleep, mood, heart rate, and state of arousal. It runs on autopilot until we become conscious of the need to act, i.e., eat, drink, urinate, remove our sweater, and so forth. Many children lack efficient interoception and, for example, may not sense when they are hungry or need to have a bowel movement.

- The vestibular sense, providing information about the position of our head in relation to the surface of the earth, the movement of our body through space, and balance. Sensations come through the inner ear. (See Chapter Four.)

- The proprioceptive sense, or proprioception, providing information about body position and movement of our body parts. Information comes from stretching and contracting our muscles. (See Chapter Five.)

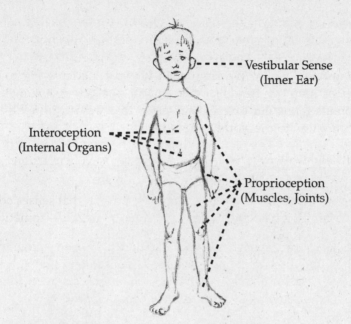

The Internal (Body-Centered) Senses

Dr. Ayres highlighted the importance of the tactile, vestibular, and proprioceptive senses that provide the sense of oneself in the world. Fundamental for functioning, these three senses lay the groundwork for a child's healthy development. When they operate automatically and efficiently, the child can turn his eyes, ears, and attention to the external world.

Typically, a child is born with his sensory apparatus intact, ready to begin his lifelong work of sensory processing.

WHAT IS SENSORY PROCESSING?

Sensory processing is the neurological procedure of organizing the information we take in from our bodies and the world around us for use in daily life. Sensory processing is dynamic, ceaseless, and cyclical. It occurs in the nervous system, which consists of 100 billion neurons, a spinal cord, and a brain. (See Appendix A.)

According to Dr. Ayres, "Over 80 percent of the nervous system is involved in processing or organizing sensory input, and thus the brain is primarily a sensory processing machine." When our brain efficiently processes sensations, we respond automatically with adaptive responses that help us master our environment. Adaptive responses are actions or thoughts that help us meet new challenges and learn new lessons. When we feel safe and need not put every effort into staying alive, we can use sensations to get on with the everyday human occupations of moving, learning, playing, working, and enjoying relationships with others.

Sensory processing involves reception, detection, integration, modulation, discrimination, postural responses, and praxis. These processes are simultaneous. Here are the basics, in an extremely simplified discussion of an extremely complex process.

Reception and Detection

One process is sensory reception. Every minute of every day, millions of sensations are received in the peripheral nervous system (PNS)—the nervous system outside the spinal cord and brain, where nerves begin and end. ("Peripheral" literally means "carried around," i.e., away from the center.) Sensations from the skin, muscles, ears, eyes, mouth, and nose travel through the PNS to the CNS. Imagine the incoming sensations saying, "Knock, knock! Here we are!"

In the process of detection, the CNS notices these sensory messages. The brain says, "Come in, all you sensations! I can see (hear, touch, smell, etc.) you!"

Integration

Integration is the continuous part of the process whereby sensations from one or more sensory systems connect in the brain.

"Meet the gang!" the brain says to the various sensations. "Touch, team up with Vision. Hearing, connect with Movement." The more sensory systems involved, the more accurate and multidimensional the information will be—and the more efficient the person's adaptive response will be.

Modulation

Another component of sensory processing is modulation. This is the term used to describe the brain's regulation of sensory input. Modulation instantly adjusts and balances the flow of sensory information into the CNS. The sensory systems need to work in tandem to keep us in sync.

Incoming sensations activate sensory receptors in a process called excitation. Excitation promotes connections between sensory input and behavioral output. Excitation is alerting. "Pay attention!" the sensations insist.

Most of the time, we do pay attention to meaningful sensory messages. If moving rhythmically in a rocking chair is calming, our brain gives us the go-ahead to continue. If spinning in circles makes us feel sick, our brain usually directs us to stop.

Sensations advising us that we are in danger are highly significant. We are hardwired to regulate our attention to danger signals in order to defend ourselves. Like all creatures, the human baby is born with sensory wariness, which he needs for survival. When potentially harmful stimuli touch him in some way, his nervous system says, "Uh, oh! Quick! Do something!"

The majority of sensations, however, are irrelevant. In a process called inhibition, our brain allows us to filter out useless information and focus on what matters at the moment. Without inhibition, we would be extremely distractible, giving full attention to every sensation, useful or not. For instance, it is unnecessary to respond to the sensation of air on our skin or of a shift in balance when we take a step, so we learn to ignore the messages. The brain says, "Settle down. That's nothing to get excited about. Don't even think about it."

HOW MODULATION AFFECTS
A CHILD'S BEHAVIOR

A Child with Typical Modulation	A Child with Sensory Modulation Disorder
During recess, Mandy, seven, plays jacks and ignores the cold pavement because the game interests her. Her hands are cold, though, so she doesn't play well. The first time she fails to scoop up the jacks, she's disappointed. The second time, she's annoyed. The third time, she's thoroughly frustrated. She says, "I'm going to jump rope." Jumping for a few minutes warms her up and makes her feel better. After recess, Mandy returns to her classroom and is calm and attentive until lunchtime.	Beth, seven, is playing jacks. She can't concentrate because the cold pavement distracts her. On her first two turns, she has trouble scooping up the jacks. Beth tries again, but her hands are too stiff. Suddenly, she explodes and screams, "I hate jacks!" She jumps to her feet, kicks the jacks into the grass, and leans against the building, crying uncontrollably. Unhappy for the rest of the morning, she can't calm down to attend to the reading lesson, and she refuses to eat lunch.

Some messages are unimportant now, although they initially grabbed our attention. After a while, when we have become accustomed to familiar messages, habituation occurs. This process tunes sensations out because they are no longer extraordinary. At first, we sense the tautness of the seat belt and the tartness of the lemon drop—and then get used to it.

Habituation does not occur readily for everyone. A process called sensitization may be the norm for sensory-sensitive people. Their brain interprets stimuli as important, unfamiliar or harmful, even if the stimuli are unimportant, familiar, and benign. Quicker and longer than other people, they notice sensations and are bothered or distracted by them. Always, the seat belt feels too tight and the lemon drop tastes too tart.

Here is an example to illustrate modulation: Imagine turning on the gas jet to warm the tea kettle. At first, you turn the dial a bit too far, too fast, and the gas leaps high. If you keep the dial there, the water will quickly come to a boil. But if you twist the dial back to inhibit the gas, the gas will calm down and heat the water at a moderate pace. You have modulated the amount and intensity of fire.

When excitation and inhibition are balanced, we can make smooth transitions from one state to another. Thus, we can switch gears from inattention to attention, from sulks to smiles, from drowsiness to alertness, and from relaxation to readiness for action. Modulation determines how efficiently we self-regulate, in every aspect of our lives.

Sensory Discrimination

Another aspect of sensory processing is discrimination, the ability to tell the difference among and between sensory stimuli. Discrimination has to do with the temporal and spatial characteristics of sensations—that is, with characteristics of timing and space.

Say you are on the beach, playing Frisbee with your child. The Frisbee flies through the air. With good sensory discrimination, you perceive it coming toward you, judge how fast it is approaching and where it is in space, and run at the right pace to the right place to catch it. "Aha!" the brain says as it processes all that Frisbee information. "I know what this means and just how to respond!"

Sensory discrimination allows us to perceive:

• Qualities of sensations—How fast am I moving? Where am I? Is my voice loud? Are my shoes tight? Is this bucket heavy? Is that snow cold?

• Similarities of sensations—Have I heard that song before? Does "four" rhyme with "door" . . . or with "five"? Is my right arm stretched as high as my left arm? Does this rabbit feel like my cat?

• Differences among sensations—Is this sound I hear "cot" or "cog"? Is that symbol a Stop sign or a Yield sign? Which train is moving—the one I'm on or the one on the next track?

Sensory discrimination develops with neurological maturation. As a child matures, he responds less self-protectively to every sensation and becomes more discriminatory about what is happening in his body and the environment. He learns to use sensations for organized behavior. For instance, when Granny arrives at the door, the child runs for a hug because integrated sensations about what he has seen, whom he has touched, and how he has moved through space teach him how to respond.

Please note: Discrimination should take precedence over defensiveness in everyday situations. Of course, at any age, a person

HOW SENSORY DISCRIMINATION TAKES PRECEDENCE OVER SENSORY DEFENSIVENESS AS CHILDREN MATURE

Child's Age	Growing Importance of Discrimination
Infant: Defensiveness is foremost.	Defensive .... Discriminative
Toddler: Defensiveness and discrimination level off.	Defensive .... Discriminative
Kindergartner: Discrimination is foremost.	Discriminative .... Defensive

can always revert to defensiveness when a true threat occurs, for this capability diminishes but does not disappear.

The chart on page 60 gives a general picture of how this shift occurs as the child develops.

Sensory-Based Motor Skills

In a nanosecond, the CNS receives, detects, integrates, modulates, and discriminates incoming sensory messages. The end result of sensory processing is when the brain sends outgoing messages that prepare the person to do something. Immediately, the brain says, "OK, let's move!" (Or, "Let's act! Let's not act! Let's think! Let's pay attention! Let's talk, cry, or giggle!")

For instance, when motor output goes to the arms, legs, eyes, and other body parts, it prepares the child to move in a satisfying way that encourages her to do more and to do it better. Motor output involves postural responses and praxis.

POSTURAL RESPONSES

Efficient sensory processing is necessary for normal movement. Equipped with the sensory information he needs, the child has good postural responses and bilateral coordination.

Postural responses extend the child's trunk, neck, and head upward, against the pull of gravity. His equilibrium and bilateral coordination allow him to experiment with different movements and positions. The child can get into and stay in a stable position. He can get into an unstable position, too, such as leaning over to retrieve a dropped pencil, and then regain his balance.

With firm muscle tone, he bends and straightens his muscles to stretch and reach. He grasps, turns, and releases objects such as spoons and doorknobs. He gets on a swing and, in Dr. Ayres' words, can "hold on and stay put." He enjoys different kinds of weight-bearing movement, such as crawling and doing push-ups. Changing positions smoothly, he shifts his weight from foot to foot, or rotates body parts, whipping his arms around his torso like a flag on a pole.

The child maintains his balance and upright position when

standing or sitting. He uses both sides of the body together to catch a ball, watch a bird fly, and jump with both feet. He uses one side alone to kick a ball, and, by the age of four or five, writes with a preferred hand.

Good postural responses contribute to the child's confidence that he can control his body and master new challenges.

PRAXIS

How do you learn to run, skip, type, flip pancakes, or use a digital camera? How do you get to Carnegie Hall?

Praxis, praxis, praxis!

Praxis (Greek for "doing, action, practice") is based partly on efficient, unconscious sensory processing and partly on conscious thought. It is a broad term denoting coordinated and voluntary action. (The term "motor planning" is often used as a synonym for praxis.) Praxis is the ability:

1) To ideate, or conceptualize, an unfamiliar and complicated action involving several steps,

2) To organize one's body to carry out the motor plan, and

3) To execute, or carry out, the plan, or at least make some progress.

Praxis permits us to do what we need and want to do as we go about our occupations of daily living. Thanks to praxis, we can pump on a swing and pump gas, write in cursive and line up a column of numbers, grind pepper and punch the right elevator button, suck poppy seeds from our teeth and whistle "Dixie."

The child is not born with praxis. Praxis is a learned skill. The child develops it over time as she touches and explores objects and learns to move her body in different ways. Each time she rehearses ordinary actions such as handing out cupcakes, zipping her jacket, and organizing her backpack, her motor planning skills improve.

Mastering one motor skill leads to trying another that is more challenging. The more the child does, the more she can do. For instance, after gaining confidence on a jungle gym, a child may use her skills to climb a tree or hang upside down from a monkey bar. This is an example of adaptive behavior.

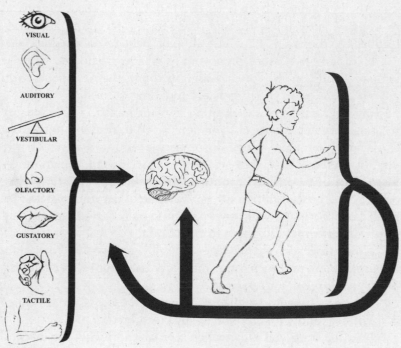

VISUAL

AUDITORY

VESTIBULAR

OLFACTORY

GUSTATORY

TACTILE

PROPRIOCEPTIVE

The Process of Sensory Input, Organization, Motor Output and Continual Feedback

Adapted with permission from Anita C. Bundy and Jane Koomar: "Orchestrating intervention: The art of practice," in Bundy, A.C., Lane, S.J., and Murray, E.A.: *Sensory Integration: Theory and Practice,* 2nd ed. (2002). Philadelphia: F.A. Davis, p. 256.

Sensory Processing Working As It Should

In a nutshell, sensory processing involves input, organization, and output. Sensory input is the neurological process of receiving messages from receptors inside and on the surface of the body. In the next step, the brain organizes the sensations. In the motor output part of the process, the brain sends out instructions to the body so the person can do what she wants to do—run, play, climb, talk, eat, sleep, and so forth. As the person engages in all these human activities, the movement of the body and the doing of the activity lead to more sensory input through the sensory receptors and more feedback to the brain. The illustration on page 63 shows this cycle.

Here is how sensory processing works as it should: Suppose you are sitting on the couch, leafing through the newspaper. You pay no attention to the upholstery touching your skin, or the car passing by outside, or the position of your hands. These sensory messages are irrelevant, and you don't need to respond to them.

Then your child plops down beside you and says, "I love you." Simultaneously, your senses of sight, hearing, touch, movement, and body position (and maybe smell, too) are stimulated. Sensory receptors throughout your peripheral nervous system take in all this information and sweep it into your central nervous system. The information zooms to your brain.

Now, these sensory messages are relevant. Swiftly, your brain organizes them and then sends messages back out so you can produce a sensory-motor response.

You respond with language: "I love you, too."

You respond with emotion: a gush of affection.

And, because you know where you are and where your child is, you know how much time it will take to get to her. Anticipating how much force to use for a "feel good" hug, you respond with movement. You drop the newspaper, lean over, open your arms, and embrace your child.

No one part of the central nervous system works alone. Messages must go back and forth from one part to another. When sensory messages come in and motor messages go out in a synchronized way, we can do what we need to do.

THREE EXAMPLES OF INPUT, ORGANIZATION, AND OUTPUT USED IN SMOOTH SENSORY-MOTOR RESPONSES

The Blaring Horn

SENSORY INPUT: Walking to work, you hum along to a song playing through your earphones. At an intersection, you look both ways, decide it's safe to cross, and step off the curb. Then you hear a blaring horn. Your auditory (hearing) sense receives the stimulus of the sound and sends the message to your brain.

NEUROLOGICAL ORGANIZATION: Suddenly, you stop hearing the music. Your brain has a more urgent task: to filter out all irrelevant sounds, analyze the new message, interpret the sound as a danger signal, and organize the information for use.

MOTOR OUTPUT: Your brain tells you how to react with an appropriate motor response. You do what you need to do and jump back.

The Sour Plum

SENSORY INPUT: You see a plum that looks juicy, ripe and sweet. You bite into it and discover that your expectation was wrong; it's sour. Your gustatory (taste) sense sends the message to your brain.

NEUROLOGICAL ORGANIZATION: Your brain interprets "sour" as harmful and organizes the sensory message for use.

MOTOR OUTPUT: Your brain tells the muscles in your mouth how to respond. You spit out the morsel and tell yourself to check more carefully the next time.

The Tilting Chair

SENSORY INPUT: Seaside, you lower yourself into a folding aluminum chair. The chair's back legs plunge into the sand. Unexpectedly, you tip backwards.

NEUROLOGICAL ORGANIZATION: Your brain analyzes this loss of equilibrium.

MOTOR OUTPUT: Your brain instructs you to protect yourself. Your core muscles contract, your head cranes forward and your hands grab the armrests. You regain your balance before tumbling backwards and upside down into the sand.

The more efficient our brain is at processing sensory input, the more effective our behavioral output will be. The more effective our output, the more feedback we receive to help us take in new sensory information and continue life-sustaining, never-ending sensory processing.

THE TYPICAL DEVELOPMENT OF SENSORY PROCESSING IN INFANTS AND CHILDREN

Becoming functional is a developmental process. It evolves as the maturing child builds his sense of self.

Dr. Ayres used a diagram to show four levels of sensory development. Her concept could be compared to a child's block construction. At first, the little child pushes blocks around on one level. Eventually, he figures out how to add a second level to the first. Then he adds a third level, and a fourth.

Sensory processing builds the same way. Each level rests on the building blocks laid down before. Just as the top level of the child's

A Variation of Dr. Ayres's "Four Levels of Sensory Integration"

Level One: Primary Sensory Systems
Touch
Balance & Movement
Body Position
(Other senses)

Level Two: Sensory-Motor Skills
Body Awareness
Use of Both Sides of Body
Hand Preference
Motor Planning

Level One: Primary Sensory Systems
Touch
Balance & Movement
Body Position
(Other senses)

Level Three: Perceptual Motor Skills
Auditory Discrimination
Speech and Language
Visual Discrimination
Eye-hand Coordination
Purposeful Activity

Level Two: Sensory-Motor Skills
Body Awareness
Use of Both Sides of Body
Hand Preference
Motor Planning

Level One: Primary Sensory Systems
Touch
Balance & Movement
Body Position
(Other senses)

Level Four: Academic Readiness
Academic Skills
Complex Motor Skills
Regulation of Attention
Organized Behavior
Self-Esteem & Self-Control

Level Three: Perceptual Motor Skills
Auditory Discrimination
Speech and Language
Visual Discrimination
Eye-hand Coordination
Purposeful Activity

Level Two: Sensory-Motor Skills
Body Awareness
Use of Both Sides of Body
Hand Preference
Motor Planning

Level One: Primary Sensory Systems
Touch
Balance & Movement
Body Position
(Other senses)

block building needs support, so his readiness for complex skills rests on the foundation of the tactile, vestibular, and proprioceptive senses. (See Appendix B for a discussion of the four levels.)

By the time a child is ready for preschool, the blocks for complex skill development should be in place. What are these blocks?

• Ability to modulate touch sensations through the skin, especially unexpected, light touch, and to discriminate among the physical properties of objects by touching them (tactile sense),

• Ability to adjust one's body to changes in gravity, and to feel comfortable moving through space (vestibular sense),

• Ability to be aware of one's body parts (proprioceptive sense),

• Ability to use the two sides of the body in a cooperative manner (bilateral coordination), and

• Ability to interact successfully with the physical environment; to plan, organize, and carry out a sequence of unfamiliar actions; to do what one needs and wants to do (praxis).

Every child has an appetite for sensory nourishment. Inner drive, or self-motivation, urges him to participate actively in experiences that promote sensory processing. In daily life, he explores the environment, tries new activities, and strives to meet increasingly complex challenges. Mastering each new challenge makes him feel successful, and success gives him the confidence to forge ahead.

So, What *Is* Sensory Processing Disorder?

Sensory Processing Disorder is difficulty in the way the brain takes in, organizes and uses sensory information, causing a person to have problems interacting effectively in the everyday environment.

Sensory stimulation may cause difficulty in one's movement, emotions, attention, or adaptive responses. SPD is an umbrella term covering several distinct disorders that affect how the child uses his senses.

Having SPD does not imply brain damage or disease, but rather what Dr. Ayres called "indigestion of the brain," or a "traffic jam in the brain." Here is what may happen:

- The child's CNS may not receive or detect sensory information.

- The brain may not integrate, modulate, organize, and discriminate sensory messages efficiently.

- The disorganized brain may send out inaccurate messages to direct the child's actions. Deprived of the accurate feedback he needs to behave in a purposeful way, he may have problems in looking and listening, paying attention, interacting with people and objects, processing new information, remembering, and learning.

Pinpointing a person's specific type of SPD matters greatly in order to decide upon the most appropriate treatment. (See Chapter Eight). The categories of Sensory Modulation Disorder, Sensory Discrimination Disorder, and Sensory-Based Motor Disorder—mentioned in Chapter One—are explained more fully here.

Sensory Modulation Disorder

A common problem among children with SPD is Sensory Modulation Disorder (SMD). This is a problem of timing in the CNS. Inhibition must be timed just right to balance excitation, so that simultaneous sensory messages can be synchronized.

A child with quick or intense inhibition has a low threshold for sensations, whether they are meaningful or meaningless, positive or negative. He's the tea kettle with the gas turned up too high. Sensations "pour on the heat," activating all his receptors. He responds to them all, roiling and boiling, bubbling over. He needs help to simmer down.

A child with slow inhibition has a high threshold for sensations. She's the tea kettle with the gas turned too low; she is not receiving enough heat to get activated. She needs help to light her fire.

What happens when a child's nervous system has a problem with modulation? The child may be overresponsive, underresponsive, sensory seeking, or have a combination, with fluctuating responsivity. All of these problems interfere with the child's interactions at home, at school and in the community. He needs guidance to help him "come to the table," be part of the family or classroom team, and engage in active, meaningful play.

SENSORY OVERRESPONSIVITY: THE SENSORY AVOIDER—"OH, NO!"

The most frequently seen type of a sensory modulation problem is overresponsivity to sensations coming from one or several systems. (Synonymous terms are hypersensitivity, hyperresponsiveness, hyperreactivity, oversensitivity and sensory defensiveness.) Overresponsivity to touch stimuli and sounds is common and often referred to as "tactile defensiveness" and "auditory defensiveness." "Sensory defensiveness" is the term used when all the senses are affected.

The overresponsive child's brain cannot inhibit sensations efficiently. He may be quite distractible because he is paying attention to all stimuli, even if the stimuli are not useful. Overaroused and unable to screen the irrelevant from the relevant, he seeks to defend himself from most sensations. He may respond as if they were irritating, annoying, or even threatening.

Most people alert to a novel sensory experience—say to a light touch or a lump in the mashed potatoes—and then shrug it off, but this child cannot let it go. Instead of responding with a typical, "Uh, oh, what's that?" he may respond with, "Oh, no! Don't do this to me!" Most people respond to a scary situation—say, a bumblebee or angry shouts—with a fight, flight, freeze, or fright response, eventually calming down, but this sensory avoider goes to extremes.

How does his fight, flight, freeze, or fright response play out? If "fight" is his modus operandi, he responds with vigorous resistance or hostility. He may be negative and defiant, lashing out.

If "flight" is his manner, he reacts with an aversive response. An aversive response is a feeling of revulsion and repugnance toward a sensation, accompanied by an intense desire to avoid or turn away from it. The child may actively withdraw, fleeing from sensations by running away, jumping back, hiding under the table, climbing on furniture or trying to claw his way out, desperate to get away from perceived threats.

Or, he may "flee" by withdrawing passively, simply avoiding the people and objects that distress him. He never gets close to them, or he walks away. Often, adults think he avoids mud pies and merry-go-rounds because "those just aren't his thing." In fact, he may yearn to participate in the activities his classmates enjoy, but just can't.

If "freeze" is his style, he may stop in his tracks, unable to move, speak, or even breathe.

If "fright" is his way, then the world is a scary place. Everything may make him crumple and cry. Or he may be fearful and cautious, closing out unfamiliar people and situations.

However possible, he will avoid sensations, particularly touch and movement experiences, because he can't tolerate them. He may misinterpret a casual touch as a life-threatening blow, feel that he will fall off the face of the earth if he is nudged, or be distressed by changes in routine, loud noises, and crowded settings.

For the out-of-sync child with overresponsivity, meltdowns are common. They may be frequent, happening several times a day. They may be intense, emotional and loud. They may last a long time, perhaps hours or all day. They may be "off the scale," going far, far beyond other children's responses to the same situation.

The child may have difficulty understanding gestural communication, too. He may overreact to nonverbal cues and respond with anxiety or hostility. He may be extremely sensitive to someone else's displeasure, even if the displeasure is not directed toward him.

SENSORY UNDERRESPONSIVITY:
THE SENSORY DISREGARDER—"HO, HUM"

Underresponsivity to sensations is another type of SMD. (Other terms are hyporesponsiveness, hyporeactivity, hyposensitivity and undersensitivity.)

The child reacts less intensely to sensations than do typically developing children. This sensory disregarder needs a lot of stimulation just to achieve ordinary arousal or alertness. His response to the world is "Ho, hum."

The child may be one of two types or sensory disregarders. He may be withdrawn and difficult to engage. Or, he may be so gifted and creative that he does notice sensory stimuli because he is self-absorbed and preoccupied with intellectual pursuits. Determining the underlying cause of a child's problem is essential, and a therapist's art and science are required to figure it out.

The sensory disregarder may appear to be a "space cadet" or "out to lunch." He may be passive, lack initiative and unable to get going. He may tire easily and seem sleepy, and as a baby, he may have slept and slept and slept.

Also, the sensory disregarder may eat and eat and eat, perhaps unaware that he is full. A solution for the child who tends to keep eating is to give him water, soup, or fresh fruit to fill him up before meals and to serve smaller portions.

The underresponsive child may miss cues that other children catch easily. He may bump into desks and people because he doesn't perceive them in time to move aside. He may hurt himself because he doesn't register "hot" or "sharp" as painful sensations. He may chew on inedible objects, such as shirt cuffs and toys, to get sensory information through his mouth.

The child may have trouble understanding gestural communication. He may misinterpret nonverbal cues and respond slowly to unspoken messages. He may not "read" other people's facial expressions and body language. He may not laugh at a clown's antics, may not comprehend that the teacher is beckoning the children to go indoors, and may not respond to a person's frown or an animal's growl.

SENSORY SEEKING:
THE SENSORY CRAVER—"MORE, MORE!"

The sensory-seeking child craves more stimulation than other children and never seems to get enough. "More, more, more!" he cries. He needs it and likes it. He may be a "toucher and feeler" and a "bumper and crasher." His brain and body are telling him that he must act, but he often acts in a disorganized way.

He likes to burp and flatulate, talk and hum. He may chew on his fingers and shirt cuffs and collar for extra input.

He craves movement and seeks vigorous experiences, such as spinning for exceptionally long times on the tire swing. Often, he will not feel dizzy. He may get into upside-down positions, with his head hanging over the mattress. He is a climber—on the monkey bars at the playground and on the bookshelf, the window sill and the car roof. Another characteristic of the sensory craver is that he may seek one kind of sensation, but pay scant attention to others.

Busy TV screens may attract him, as may strobe lights, loud noises, crowds, and places with plenty of action, such as football games and car races. He may sniff food, people, and objects, seeking strong odors that others find objectionable. He may crave four-alarm chili, spicy Chinese food, pickles and pickle juice, lemons and red-hot candy.

This child is often a risk taker and a daredevil and may also have poor impulse control. No wonder others frequently look upon him as a troublemaker.

SENSORY COMBINATION: THE SENSORY FLUCTUATOR—"I LOVE THIS, I HATE THAT."

Another possible type of sensory modulation disorder is a combination of overresponsivity and underresponsivity as the child's brain rapidly shifts back and forth. Fluctuating responsivity interferes with the child's adaptive responses. She may be overly sensitive to some sensations, yet shrug off others. She may crave movement, yet cringe from messy play. How common it is to be not all one way!

This sensory fluctuator may seek intense sensory experiences—such as spinning on playground equipment—but be unable to tolerate them. Or, she may seek intense experiences some days and avoid them on other days. Her on-again-off-again responses may depend on the time of day, the place, what she ate, how much sleep she had, and the kind of sensory stimuli. Her behavior implies that her nervous system is undecided, saying, "I love this, I hate that."

Her behavior bewilders the adults who care for her. Sometimes she will seem to be in sync, sometimes she won't. Her attention span for things she enjoys may be excellent until certain sensations get in her way. This child is particularly challenging to raise and to teach because it is so hard to know how and when to help her.

The child has great difficulty functioning in daily life. She is not on an even keel and becomes easily upset. Once upset, she may have difficulty recovering.

She may be well regulated at home but have problems at school, or vice versa. She may feel safe and in control at one place, but uncertain and out of control in another. The need to feel in control of people, objects, and experiences is a major issue for the child who does not feel in control of herself.

Sensory Discrimination Disorder

THE SENSORY JUMBLER—"HUH?"

The child with sensory discrimination disorder has difficulty differentiating among and between stimuli. His CNS inaccurately processes sensations, so he is unable to use the information to make purposeful, adaptive responses and function throughout the day. He misgauges the importance of objects and experiences. He may not "get" sensory messages that others use to protect themselves, to learn about their environment, and to relate successfully to other people.

The child often has significant difficulty with visual-spatial tasks. He may be unable to judge where objects and people are in space and may miss important visual cues on the page and in social interactions. He often has auditory discrimination problems, too. These cause him to be easily confused by similar sounding words or by verbal instructions.

This sensory jumbler may have poor body awareness, falling frequently and having trouble catching himself. He uses inappropriate force when using pencils, manipulating toys, and playing with other children. He breaks pencils, struggles to fit Legos together, and bumps into people and things because he is not paying attention.

When the sensory jumbler has problems with touch, movement, and body position, he often has dyspraxia, too. That is no surprise, as praxis requires a discriminatory sense of how one's body works.

Sensory-Based Motor Disorders

In addition to modulation and discrimination problems, a child with SPD may have sensory-based problems that affect how she moves.

POSTURAL DISORDER:
THE SENSORY SLUMPER—"DON'T WANT TO."

Postural Disorder causes the child to have poor posture. She may have low muscle tone and be "loose and floppy." She slouches while sitting or standing and slumps over the desk and dining room table. This droopy child is besieged by the "gravity monster." The reason may be the inefficient sensory processing of vestibular and proprioceptive sensations about where her body is in space and what it is doing.

According to Dr. Ayres, "The major symptoms manifested by children with this type of dysfunction . . . are related to the fact that man is a bilateral and symmetrical being." When a child has not developed a sense of two-sidedness, Postural Disorder may interfere with nature's plan, which is to keep upright and ready to spring into action, using both sides of the body together or separately as needed.

The child may have a problem with bilateral integration, the neurological process of connecting sensations from both sides of the body. The result is poor bilateral coordination, the ability to use both sides of the body together. For instance, she may struggle to gallop, skip, or pedal a bicycle.

She may have difficulties positioning her body and maintaining her equilibrium. Getting into different positions, such as kneeling or stretching to her tiptoes, without tipping over may also be a challenge.

Often the child will have poor ocular (eye movement) control, affecting binocularity—the use of both eyes together as a team. This will hinder depth perception, body movement, motor planning, and reaching for objects. A problem with crossing the midline, i.e., using the eye, hand or foot of one side of the body in the space of the other eye, hand, or foot, may interfere with her ease in painting a horizon at the easel or swinging a baseball bat.

Keeping up with her peers wears her out. Her grasp on doorknobs and faucets, toys and lunchboxes, is weak. When she sits on the floor, her legs are often in the "W" position, with her knees pointing forward and feet splayed to the side for added stability.

Flexing and extending her muscles, shifting her weight from one foot to the other, twisting her body around while planted on two feet, moving like animals, and so forth, are movement activities that we expect children to enjoy. For the sensory slumper, they are often too daunting.

DYSPRAXIA: THE SENSORY FUMBLER—
"I CAN'T DO THAT."

Dyspraxia is the second type of Sensory-Based Motor Disorder. Dyspraxia refers to disruption in sensory processing and motor planning in children who are still developing.

Dyspraxia causes children to be clumsy and ineffective in their actions. They cannot organize their bodies to move. They reach for a stair tread or a soda can and they miss—a problem called "motor overshoot." Dr. Ayres says that "these children may have normal intelligence and muscles. The problem is in the 'bridge' between their intellect and their muscles." For some reason, accurate information about touch, movement, and body position cannot cross that bridge from the brain to the body, so the child does not "get it" and cannot use it. (Many examples of how sensory dysfunction leads to Dyspraxia are in the next chapters.)

SIX IMPORTANT CAVEATS

In this book, you will find many checklists of characteristics of children with SPD. You will also find numerous examples of out-of-sync behavior that illustrate the various ways SPD plays out at home and school. You may say, "Eureka! This is my child, to a tee!" On the other hand, you may say, "This is definitely not my child, because my child doesn't have all these symptoms." Perhaps your child is somewhere in between.

As you read along, please remember the following caveats:

1) The child with SPD does not exhibit every characteristic mentioned in this book. SPD is not one but several disorders, and nobody can have them all.

2) The child with SPD usually has difficulties in more than one sense, but she may have a concentration of problems in one system, such as the tactile system. If so, she will not

necessarily exhibit every characteristic of that category. Thus, the child with vestibular dysfunction may have poor balance but good muscle tone; the child with tactile dysfunction may find light touch intolerable but be a good eater.

3) The child may be both overresponsive and under-responsive in one sensory system, or may be overresponsive to one kind of sensation and underresponsive to another, or may respond differently to the same stimulus depending on the time and context, fluctuating back and forth. Yesterday, after a long recess, he may have coped well with a fire alarm; today, when recess is cancelled, he may have a meltdown when a door clicks shut. Context makes a huge difference.

4) Categories of SPD are not always clear-cut and often overlap. Sensory Overresponsivity and Sensory Under-responsivity, for instance, often look like and merge with Sensory Discrimination Disorder and Dyspraxia.

5) The child may exhibit characteristics of a sensory disorder, yet have another disorder altogether. For example, the child who typically withdraws from being touched may seem to have tactile overresponsivity but instead may have a childhood anxiety disorder or may have been abused.

6) Everyone has some sensory processing problems now and then, because we are all on the sensory processing continuum and no one is well-regulated all the time. All kinds of stimuli can temporarily disrupt functioning of the brain, either by too much or too little sensory stimulation.

COMPARISON OF
TYPICAL SENSORY PROCESSING
AND SENSORY PROCESSING DISORDER

	Typical Sensory Processing	*Sensory Processing Disorder*
What:	The ability to take in sensory information from one's body and the environment, to organize this information, and to use it to function in daily life.	The ineffective processing of tactile, vestibular, and/or proprioceptive sensations. The person may have difficulty with other basic senses, too.
Where:	Occurs in the central nervous system (nerves, spinal cord, and brain), in a well balanced, reciprocal process.	Occurs in the central nervous system, where the flow between sensory input and motor output is disrupted.
Why:	To enable a person to survive, to make sense of the world, and to interact with the environment in meaningful ways.	Neuronal connections in the central nervous system are ineffective.
How:	Happens automatically as the person takes in sensations through sensory receptors in the skin, the inner ear, the muscles, and the eyes, ears, mouth, and nose.	Sensory neurons do not send effective messages into the central nervous system, and/or motor neurons do not send effective messages out to the body for adaptive behavioral responses.
When:	Begins *in utero* and continues developing throughout childhood, with most functions established by adolescence.	Occurs before, during, or shortly after birth.

Chapter Three

HOW TO TELL IF YOUR CHILD HAS A PROBLEM WITH THE TACTILE SENSE

THREE KINDERGARTNERS AT CIRCLE TIME

The kindergartners are gathering for circle time. In the center of the rug, Miss Baker has arranged a variety of squashes: acorn, butternut, patty pan, pumpkin, summer, and zucchini.

Most of the children sit down on their individual carpet squares. Robert, however, stands aside and waits until the others are seated. Then he gingerly picks up his carpet square and moves it toward the wall. He pulls two plastic dinosaurs from his pocket and grips one in each hand. Finally, he sits down, as far as possible from Lena, his nearest neighbor.

Patrick finds his carpet square, but, instead of sitting, he makes a crash landing, sprawling face down on the rug. He spreads his arms and legs and swishes them on the rug, shouting, "Look! I'm a windshield wiper!"

Miss Baker says, "Please sit up in your own space, Patrick."

He sits up and begins to wrestle with another boy until

Miss Baker says, "Please keep your hands to yourself, Patrick."

Eventually, circle time begins. Miss Baker passes each squash around the circle, so the children can get a feel for them.

Patrick squeezes every squash when he gets his hands on it. He rolls the summer squash between his hands and rubs it down his legs. He licks the acorn squash and bites the zucchini.

Miss Baker reminds him, "Just use your hands, not your mouth. And please pass the squash to Lena. It's her turn."

Lena, however, is not paying attention. She gazes out the window. When Patrick flings each squash into her lap, she looks down in surprise. Without examining the squashes, she passes them quickly to Robert.

But Robert refuses to touch the vegetables. When Lena offers him the first squash, he jabs his dinosaurs toward her face.

Lena recoils and drops the squash. Having figured that Robert isn't receptive, she places the subsequent samples in front of him.

Using his dinosaurs, Robert pushes each squash away.

Miss Baker lines up the squashes in the center of the rug. She says, "Now, look at the squashes. What can you tell me about them?"

Several children volunteer their observations: "The pumpkin is heavy." "The zucchini is smooth." "The patty pan has a bumpy edge."

Miss Baker says, "You are good observers! What about you, Lena? Do you have something to add?"

Lena hesitates. Then she says, "I see six."

"True!" says Miss Baker. "Anything else?"

"Nothing," Lena says.

Miss Baker turns to Robert and says, "How about you?"

Robert says, "This is boring."

"This isn't boring!" Patrick bellows. He lunges forward, scoops all the squashes into a pile, and rolls on top of them. "This is fun!"

Miss Baker extricates the squashes from Patrick and says, "Let's put the squashes away now and sing a song. Then it's time for free play in the classroom."

Circle time comes to a close.

Atypical Patterns of Behavior

To the casual observer, Robert, Patrick, and Lena may seem like typical preschoolers. It's easy to look at their behavior and say, "That's just the way they are." But if we look closer, we may notice atypical patterns of behavior.

Touching and being touched distress Robert. He avoids being near the other children and defends himself with his dinosaurs. Handling his carpet square is unpleasant. He refuses to touch the squashes with his hands.

Touching and being touched delight Patrick. He uses his whole body to feel the rug. He tackles another child. He manhandles, mouths, and rolls on the squashes.

Touching objects to learn about them is not Lena's forte. Giving scant attention to the squashes, she doesn't perceive whether they are heavy or light, big or small, bumpy or smooth. Her only observation is about their quantity, not their quality.

These children may appear to be very different, but they have something in common: an identifiable problem with the tactile sense.

On the next pages you will learn how the tactile sense is supposed to function, followed by an explanation of the types of SPD that affect Robert, Patrick, and Lena.

THE SMOOTHLY FUNCTIONING
TACTILE SENSE

The tactile system, or sense of touch, plays a major part in determining physical, mental, and emotional human behavior. Every one of us, from infancy onward, needs constant tactile stimulation to keep us organized and functioning.

We get tactile information through sensory receiving cells—called receptors—in our skin, from head to toe. Touch sensations of light touch, deep pressure, skin stretch, vibration, movement, temperature, and pain activate tactile receptors. These sensations are external and come from stimuli outside our body.

We are always actively touching or passively being touched by something—other people, furniture, clothes, spoons. Even if we are stark naked, our feet still touch the ground, and the air touches our skin.

According to Dr. Ayres, "Touch is one of the senses that is especially involved in the ongoing process contributing to perception of other types of sensation. Touch has been one of the predominating senses throughout evolution, is a predominant sensation at birth, and probably continues to be more critical to human function throughout life than is generally recognized."

This huge sensory system connects us to the world and bonds us to others, starting when we first nestle at our mother's breast, skin to skin. It gives us essential information for body awareness, motor planning, visual discrimination, language, academic learning, emotional security, and social skills.

Two Components: Defensive ("Okay!" or "Uh, Oh!") and Discriminative ("Aha!")

Two components make up the tactile sense. First is the protective (or defensive) system. Its purpose is to alert us to potentially harmful—or healthful—stimuli. Tactile receptors for this protective system are especially in hairy skin on the head, face, and genitals. Light touch is the stimulus that causes these receptors to respond.

Sometimes a light touch is alarming, such as a mosquito alighting on our skin. "Uh, oh!" our nervous system tells us. We respond negatively, for self-preservation. Sometimes a light touch is charming, such as a lover's gentle caress, and our nervous system says, "Okay!" We respond positively, for preservation of the species!

Ordinarily, modulation of touch sensations improves as we interact with other people and objects. We learn to inhibit sensations that do not matter and to tolerate trifling touches that would have irritated us in infancy. Of course, when a stranger gets too close, we shrink; when a lash gets in our eye, we blink. But usually, we ignore light touch sensations because they do not grab our attention the way deep pain or extremes in temperature do.

The second component of the tactile sense teaches us to discriminate what kind of touch we are feeling. Feeling the warmth of Mommy's skin, the roughness of Daddy's stubble, the crunchiness of gravel underfoot, and the roundness of an orange, we gain conscious insights, intuition, and knowledge about the world. Where have we felt this touch before? What could that touch signify? And what should we do about it? With the capability to remember and interpret the meaning of touches, we gradually develop tactile discrimination.

"Aha!" the nervous system says, telling us:

- That we are touching something or that something is touching us,
- Where on our body the touch occurs,
- Whether the touch is light or deep, and
- How to perceive the attributes of the object, such as its size, shape, weight, density, temperature, and texture.

The receptors for tactile discrimination are in the skin, especially on the palms and fingertips, the soles of the feet, and the mouth and tongue. Deep touch, or "touch pressure," is the stimulus that causes the receptors to respond.

As you read on, you will understand why a smoothly functioning tactile system is necessary to function normally, and how an out-of-sync tactile system is disruptive.

THE OUT-OF-SYNC TACTILE SENSE

Tactile dysfunction, a major problem, is the inefficient processing in the central nervous system of sensations perceived through the skin. All categories of SPD can interfere with the way a child organizes and uses tactile sensations.

The child has difficulty with touching, and being touched by, objects and people. He may have one or more problems with modulation, discrimination, or sensory-based motor skills as he goes through the day, depending on what subtype(s) of SPD he has. (See chart on page 10.)

Sensory Modulation Disorders

TACTILE OVERRESPONSIVITY—"OH, NO!"

The child with overresponsivity to touch (tactile defensiveness) has the tendency to respond negatively and emotionally to unexpected, light touch sensations. The child will respond this way not only to actual touch but also to the anticipation of being touched. Perceiving most touch sensations to be uncomfortable, scary, or outright terrifying, he overresponds with a fight, flight, fright, or freeze response.

He may wrestle in your arms as you try to dress or lift him. He may wriggle out of his clothes or car seat. He may kick, punch, or scream at anyone who comes too close for comfort.

HOW TACTILE OVERRESPONSIVITY
AFFECTS A CHILD'S BEHAVIOR

A Child with Typical Modulation	A Child with Overresponsivity
Getting ready for school, Daniel, three, tolerates having his father brush his hair and wash his face. He doesn't enjoy this experience, but he can adapt to it and can recover immediately. His maturing neurological system allows him to suppress a fight-or-flight response.	Getting ready for school, Will, three, flinches when his father tries to brush his hair and wash his face. He pushes his father away and cries, "You're hurting me!" Defensiveness still rules his reactions to touch, so he produces an infantile fight-or-flight response. He's upset all during breakfast.

The child may flee from contact with finger paints, pets, and people. He may find the touch of unfamiliar people to be intolerable. Or, he may withdraw passively by simply avoiding the objects and people that distress him. He never gets close to them, or he walks away.

He may be afraid and start to cry when he has to take a bath. He may stop dead in his tracks and not know what to do when his cuffs get wet at the sink.

All children need touch information to learn about the world. So how does the child with tactile defensiveness get this information? By touching!

Parents are often mystified when they learn that their child has tactile overresponsivity. They protest, "But he often asks for hugs and back rubs. He usually carries something in his hands. How can you say he has a problem with touch?"

The answer is the type of touch that the child avoids or seeks. The child typically avoids passive, unexpected, light touch, such as a gentle kiss. A kiss is irritating, and the child may try to rub it off. While the child avoids light touch, he not only accepts but also craves deep touch, like a bear hug. A hug provides firm touch and deep pressure, which feels wonderful and actually helps suppress sensitivity to light touch.

While the child may long for the hug, he may reject the hugger unless the hugger is on his "OK" list. A likely OK person is a parent or another predictable individual whom the child trusts. People on his "Not OK" list may be classmates, baby-sitters, relatives, and even loving grandparents, to their great sorrow.

This child needs touch information more than children with a well-regulated tactile sense who get it just by waking up in the morning and going through the day. To get the stimulation his brain needs, he may actively, repeatedly touch those surfaces and textures that provide soothing and comforting tactile experiences. For example, he may cling to a blanket, like Linus in the *Peanuts* comic strip. He may also hold objects such as a stick or a toy in his hand. He may mouth toys. Perhaps these objects help him defend himself from the unexpected touch sensations abounding in the environment.

TACTILE UNDERRESPONSIVITY—"HO, HUM."
The child with underresponsivity to touch tends to disregard touch, whether the touch is soothing or painful.

Instead of murmuring, "Mmm!" when his mother cradles him, he seems to say, "Ho, hum. This TLC has no effect on me." Instead of crying, "Ouch!" when he stubs his toe, he seems to say, "Ho, hum. I didn't notice."

Unlike the ever-alert, overresponsive child, the sensory disregarder may not respond to touch effectively enough to do a good job of self-protection. In fact, he may seem unaware of touch altogether, unless the touch is very intense.

HOW UNDERRESPONSIVITY
AFFECTS A CHILD'S BEHAVIOR

A Child with Typical Modulation	*A Child with Underresponsivity*
Randy, six, falls off his bicycle, scraping his knees. He runs inside and tearfully tells his baby sitter that he had a bad accident. She bandages his wounds and soothes him. Eventually, he stops crying, although he hobbles around the house and complains for a little while. As soon as his friend comes to play, he forgets about his discomfort.	Georgio, six, falls off his bicycle. He scrapes both knees, but pays little attention to his injuries. He remounts his bike and continues to ride. When his baby-sitter notices his wounds and tries to clean them, he brushes her off. "It doesn't hurt," he says.

SENSORY SEEKING—"MORE!"
All children need abundant sensations to learn about the world. The sensory craver needs more deep pressure and more skin contact than most. He may touch and feel everything in sight, running his hands over furniture and walls, and handling items that other children understand are "no-nos." Even if an object is inappropriate to handle, such as a fragile dish or hot candle, he has "gotta touch" it.

Intensely and impulsively, he may seek to touch certain

HOW SENSORY SEEKING
AFFECTS A CHILD'S BEHAVIOR

A Child with Typical Modulation	A Child with Sensory Seeking
The kindergarten teacher gathers the children around a table covered with a plastic cloth. She spurts a mound of shaving cream in front of each child. Troy, five, enjoys finger painting in the cream. He smears it around his table space and writes his name in it. When Bryce begins to bother him, he shouts, "Stop!" and moves back. He rinses his hands and finds a puzzle to do at a table far away from Bryce.	Bryce, five, adores playing in shaving cream, the teacher's smart substitute for finger paint. He smears the cream over his hands, arms, throat, and face. He begins to smear Troy, who says, "Stop! You'll get in trouble!" Bryce turns back to the table, spreading shaving cream into other children's territories. They object and the teacher comes over to intervene. He could play here all day, but his behavior is getting in everyone else's way.

surfaces and textures that are uncomfortable to others, rubbing his hands over rough tree bark and walking barefoot on gravel. He crams his mouth with food. He gets too close to other people, bumping, pawing, and touching them, although they tell him this is unwelcome. Messy play is his true love. He'll look for and find puddles, mud, clay, glue, and paint. The more, the merrier.

The sensory craver frequently gets in trouble for his insistent, persistent, tactile explorations. His constant wallowing in messy materials ruins his clothes, trashes the classroom, and repels the people around him. Of course, his motivation is not to infuriate them but to get the sensory input his nervous system needs. Of course, most people do not understand his behavior. And, of course, the child is incapable of explaining his cravings, so everyone around him gets upset and tells him he is being bad.

Therapy can help this child's nervous system to modulate touch sensations. At home and school, an approach may be to provide him with a lot of safe, appropriate, fun, and easy tactile activities. (See *The Out-of-Sync Child Has Fun* for specific suggestions.)

SENSORY COMBINATION—
"I LOVE THIS, I HATE THAT."

The sensory fluctuator may have overresponsivity and underresponsivity to sensations, like two sides of a coin. One minute, he may truly love an experience such as having his hair brushed or being cuddled, and the next minute, hate it. He may shriek with alarm when someone touches his arm, yet be indifferent to a broken collarbone. He may love jumping on the mattress and hate getting a back rub. This, but not that! That, not this!

HOW A SENSORY COMBINATION
AFFECTS A CHILD'S BEHAVIOR

A Child with Typical Modulation	A Sensory Fluctuator
Peter, ten, and his friend Cody decide to kick a can all the way home instead of riding the bus. Invigorated from the walk, the boys are now in the kitchen, twisting dough to make pretzels. Peter does this often and is comfortable getting his hands dirty; he likes to mold and sculpt the dough into animal and people shapes.	Today Cody enjoys handling the sticky pretzel dough after walking to Peter's instead of taking the bus. Everything with Peter is fun. Then Peter's sister starts to play the saxophone. The squeaky blasts irritate Cody, and suddenly the fun is over. He can't tolerate the dough on his hands another second. He runs to the sink, scrubs his hands, and rushes out without saying thank you or good-bye.

Tactile Discrimination Disorder: "Huh?"

The out-of-sync child has difficulty paying attention to the physical attributes of objects and people. If he has a modulation problem, his central nervous system is otherwise occupied. If he is a sensory avoider, his hands may "live" in his pockets, or he may keep his fingers curled to protect his sensitive palms. If he is a sensory seeker, he may handle—or mishandle—everything in sight without discrimination.

When sensory modulation is out-of-sync, then the child's discriminative system may not arise to "take charge." (The child with poor tactile discrimination often has tactile defensiveness, but this is not always the case.) With inefficient or immature discrimination, the child will have difficulty using his tactile sense for increasingly complex purposes, such as learning at school. Even when he has met building blocks or three-ring binders before, he needs to touch and handle them repeatedly to learn about their weight, texture, and shape. "Huh?" he seems to say. "What's this?"

The child may seem out of touch with his hands, using them as if they were unfamiliar appendages. He may be unable to point a finger toward the book he wants or to button a coat without looking at what he is doing. He may have difficulty learning new manual skills, exploring materials and equipment, using classroom tools, and performing ordinary tasks. If he hurts himself, he may not perceive where he hurts and whether the pain is increasing or lessening. He may not know when he is hungry or needs to urinate.

HOW TACTILE DISCRIMINATION
AFFECTS A CHILD'S BEHAVIOR

A Typical Child	*A Child with Tactile Dysfunction*
Kindergartner Ellen is making a "guitar" by pulling rubber bands over a cigar box. Tactile discrimination helps her grasp differences among the rubber bands. She chooses several with various attributes: big and small, skinny and fat, tight and loose. She stretches them over the box and arranges them carefully so they don't overlap. By strumming or plucking, she can produce a variety of pleasing sounds.	Patsy, five, grabs a huge handful of rubber bands, but she has trouble knowing which ones are more or less flexible than others. They all seem the same to her, because her tactile discrimination is inefficient. She struggles to stretch one rubber band around the cigar box and then gives up. Problems with modulation, discrimination, and dyspraxia get in her way.

HOW THE TACTILE SENSE
AFFECTS EVERYDAY SKILLS

In addition to helping us to protect ourselves, to discriminate among objects, and to accomplish what we set out to do, the tactile sense gives us information that is necessary for many kinds of everyday skills:

- Body awareness
  (Body percept)
- Praxis (Motor planning)
- Visual discrimination

- Language
- Academic learning
- Emotional security
- Social skills

Body Awareness (Body Percept)

The tactile sense, along with the proprioceptive sense, affects a person's subconscious awareness of individual body parts, and how the body parts relate to one another and to the surrounding environment. With good tactile discrimination, a child develops body awareness (body percept), which is like a map of the body, and can then move purposefully and easily. The child has a sense of where he is and what he is doing.

The child with a tactile disorder lacks good body awareness. He is uncomfortable using his body in his environment because moving means touching. He has difficulty orienting his limbs in order to get dressed. He would rather stand in a corner than risk mingling with an unpredictable group. Shifting his position may even make him conscious of how uncomfortable he is in his clothes. Better to stand very, very still, his central nervous system tells him, and avoid it all.

HOW BODY AWARENESS
AFFECTS A CHILD'S BEHAVIOR

A Typical Child	A Child with Tactile Dysfunction
In his third-grade music class, Tyler is enjoying the song, "Head and Shoulders, Knees and Toes." He likes it when the tempo speeds up, so that tapping the right body parts at the right time gets harder. Recess is after music, and Tyler slips into his jacket, zips it up, pulls on his gloves, and heads outdoors.	Roger slumps in the back row, scowling. He hates the "Head and Shoulders" song. He always gets his body parts mixed up, and he's embarrassed. Before recess, he concentrates on getting into his coat, still a difficult task. Gloves are too much trouble, so he shuffles outdoors with his hands stuck in his pockets.

Praxis (Motor Planning)

Each new sequence of movements requires praxis, or motor planning. Certainly, the first time a child climbs a jungle gym, threads a belt through loops, or says "Lollapalooza," he must plan his movements with conscious effort. With practice, he can do these actions successfully because he has integrated tactile sensations, such as the feel of jungle gym rungs under his feet and hands.

The child who feels uncomfortable in his own skin may have poor motor planning, or dyspraxia. He may move awkwardly and have difficulty planning and organizing his movements. Thus, he may shun the very activities that would improve his praxis.

For instance, if he dislikes how the monkey bars feel, he won't try to hang from them or practice the skill of traveling beneath them, one hand after the other. If touching a dandelion makes him uneasy, he won't reach to pick it. The less he does, the less he can do. In a world where "use it or lose it" is a fact of life, this child is at a loss.

HOW PRAXIS (MOTOR PLANNING) AFFECTS A CHILD'S BEHAVIOR

A Typical Child	A Child with Dyspraxia
Charley, four, arises and puts on blue jeans and a new belt, managing to buckle it all by himself. He runs downstairs. He steadies his grapefruit with one hand and spoons it with the other. Ready for school, he climbs into the car and fastens his seat belt. Arriving at school, he unsnaps his seat belt and jumps out. On the blacktop, he spots a new tricycle. It is larger than trikes he has ridden before, but he figures out how to mount it. He stretches his feet and arms to reach the pedals and handles. He takes it for a test drive, getting a feel for its new requirements.	Lars, four, arises slowly. He ignores the blue jeans and belt his mother has set out; they're too hard to put on. He struggles into his favorite sweatpants with the elasticized waist. He goes downstairs carefully: right foot first, then left, on each step. He jabs a spoon at his grapefruit, and the dish skitters across the table. When it's time to go to school, he maneuvers himself into the car and waits for his mother to buckle him in. Arriving at school, he needs a teacher to unbuckle the seat belt. Then he inches out of the car. On the blacktop, Lars heads for an old familiar tricycle. While the other kids ride in circles around him, he sits there, dangling his feet.

GROSS-MOTOR CONTROL

Praxis is necessary for two broad categories of movement, one of which is gross-motor control. Like the super highway, this is the smooth coordination of the large, or proximal, muscles, which are closest to his body core. Gross-muscle control allows a child to bend, lift, twist, and stretch, to move his body from one place to another by creeping or running, and to maneuver his hands and feet.

The child with poor tactile (and proprioceptive) processing is out of touch with his body and with objects in his world. His

HOW GROSS-MOTOR CONTROL
AFFECTS A CHILD'S BEHAVIOR

A Typical Child	A Child with Tactile Dysfunction
Hannah, ten, enjoys the fast-moving "Over and Under" game. One person holds a ball over her head and passes it to the next person, who takes the ball, bends forward, thrusts it through her legs, and passes it to the next. Moving is fun!	For Kim, ten, playing "Over and Under" is hard. Her movements are slow and awkward. The ball feels uncomfortable in her hands, and sometimes she drops it. When she slows down or interrupts the game, the other kids get angry. Movement games are no fun at all.

gross-motor skills may be delayed, making it very difficult to learn, move, and play in meaningful ways.

FINE-MOTOR CONTROL

Praxis is necessary for another category of movement: fine-motor skills, like the byroads, which a child usually refines after establishing gross-motor skills. Fine-motor control governs the precise use of small muscles in the fingers and hands, in the toes, and in the tongue, lips, and muscles of the mouth.

Because the child with tactile dysfunction often curls his hands in loose fists or jams them in his pockets to avoid touch sensations, he has difficulty manipulating ordinary tools such as eating utensils, scissors, crayons, and pencils. So much of the school day revolves around writing and other fine-motor tasks that a problem with these skills may be extremely discouraging for the older child.

This child frequently has poor self-help skills, is a messy eater, and may also have poor articulation and immature language skills. He may use more gestures than words to communicate because the fine-motor control of his tongue and lips is inadequate.

HOW FINE-MOTOR CONTROL
AFFECTS A CHILD'S BEHAVIOR

A Typical Child	A Child with Tactile Dysfunction
Today is woodworking day for Alex's preschool class. Alex sorts through the woodbin, chooses two pieces, and hammers them together to make an airplane. He takes it outside and experiments with different ways to hold and throw it. At dinner, he explains in detail how he constructed his lovely airplane, and how well it flies. Alex has good praxis.	Josh, four, wants to construct an airplane. He isn't sure how to begin, so the teacher hands him two wood pieces. He has trouble holding the hammer, so the teacher helps him. His airplane looks pretty good. Outside, he throws it to see if it will fly. It falls at his feet. Then he stands and holds it until it is time to go home. At dinner, his father asks what he did at school. Unable to express his thoughts, Josh holds up his lovely airplane for his father to see. Josh is dyspraxic.

Visual Discrimination

The tactile system plays an important part in the development of visual discrimination—the way the brain interprets what the eyes see. By touching objects, a child stores memories of their characteristics and relationships to one another. Looking at a rain puddle, for instance, he perceives that it is wet, cool, and fun to splash in, even without touching it, because he has touched puddles before.

Normally, a young child touches what he looks at and looks at what he touches. Many experiences touching objects and people are the basis for visual discrimination.

When a child's brain mismanages touch stimuli, however, he cannot integrate tactile and visual messages. Basic information eludes him about how things appear to feel. He looks but does not understand what he sees.

HOW TACTILE PROCESSING AFFECTS
A CHILD'S VISUAL DISCRIMINATION

A Typical Child	A Child with Tactile Dysfunction
The teacher hands each kindergartner a plastic shape. Each shape has different attributes. It is big or small; red, yellow, or blue; round, square, or rectangular. Then, the teacher lays a series of similar shapes on the rug and asks the children to tell her which shape on the floor matches the one in their hands. Tiffany knows the answer right away because she has handled many objects in her five years. She places her small red square next to its mate.	The teacher hands Chrissy, five, a big yellow rectangle, and Chrissy drops it into her lap. When her turn comes to match her shape with one on the floor, Chrissy is uncertain about its size and shape. She knows her colors, though. She makes a guess and puts her big yellow rectangle next to a small yellow square. A classmate points out her error, and the teacher asks him to show Chrissy how to make a correct match.

Language

The tactile sense, in a way, leads us to language. Babies depend on touch to make contact with the world. Expanding their contacts as they move around and touch things, young children absorb others' commentaries about what they are doing.

"That's a daisy. Touch it gently."

"Pull hard on that wagon. Pull, pull!"

"Give me your foot and I'll put on your shoe."

"Where's the ball? It's under the couch. Get the ball. Throw the ball to Daddy."

"Whoops! You fell down, head over heels! That was scary. Come here; I'll brush you off and make it all better."

Words become associated with actions, body parts, objects, places, people, and feelings. Thus, children learn verbs, nouns, names, prepositions, adjectives, adverbs, and labels for emotions.

HOW TACTILE PROCESSING
AFFECTS A CHILD'S LANGUAGE

A Typical Child	A Child with Tactile Dysfunction
Jeff's eighth-grade cooking class made delicious tacos last week. Today the teacher asks the students to write down the recipe to test their memory about the various steps and processes involved. Jeff writes, "Warm taco shells in preheated oven. Grate cheese. Shred lettuce. Mince chipotle chilies. Chop cilantro. Dice tomatoes and peppers. Sauté ground beef or turkey. Drain fat. Peel and slice onion, and sauté. Spread mixture on taco shells. Arrange condiments in bowls so guests can choose what they like." Etcetera.	Gavin, thirteen, enjoys eating and thought taking a cooking class as an elective would be easy, but preparing the food is hard. Dyspraxia and tactile discrimination problems cause him to fumble with the taco ingredients, measuring spoons and knives. He jumbles everything together. Now he is supposed to write down the recipe but is vague about the manual tasks involved and the words to describe them. He wishes he could prove to the teacher that his motivation to do well is high . . . but how? He writes, "Cook meat. Cut vegetables. Serve."

When the out-of-sync child's tactile experiences are limited, so are his opportunities to develop language. In addition, the child with poor tactile awareness in his mouth, lips, tongue, and jaw may have a sensory-based motor problem called oral apraxia, which affects his ability to produce and sequence sounds necessary for speech.

Academic Learning

Tactile processing has a big impact on a child's ability to learn at school. Many objects require hands-on manipulation: art and science materials, rhythm instruments, basketballs, chalk, pencils, and paper. Taking pleasure in tactile experiences leads to exploring new materials and building a base of knowledge that will continue throughout a lifetime.

A tactile disorder prevents a child from learning easily because touch sensations distract him. He may fidget when quiet is expected, complain that others are annoying him, and have trouble settling down for academic tasks.

The child misses out on learning skills requiring the purposeful use of tools such as compasses, forks, and hammers. He misses out on learning about nature, because messy, hands-on experiences are intolerable or because he can't discriminate between an acorn and a chestnut. He misses out on learning problem-solving skills, communication skills, and "people" skills.

HOW THE TACTILE SENSE
AFFECTS A CHILD'S ACADEMIC LEARNING

A Typical Child	A Child with Tactile Dysfunction
Juan, six, likes science. Today, the teacher brings several caterpillars in a glass jar. Juan knows how it feels to handle caterpillars and asks, "May I hold the one that looks soft and fuzzy?" The teacher offers him the jar. He picks out the fuzzy caterpillar and puts it on his arm. "It tickles!"	Ricardo, six, dislikes science. While the other first-graders talk about the caterpillars, Ricardo averts his gaze. He rejects the teacher's invitation to hold the jar. He squirms in his chair and sits on his hands. He hates creepy bugs.

Emotional Security

With a well-regulated nervous system, we first learn to welcome the touch of the person (usually our mother) who takes care of our basic infantile needs. Cuddling makes us feel safe.

A close physical attachment to one or two primary caregivers sets the stage for all future personal relationships. If we feel cared for and loved, our emotional base is secure, and we learn to reciprocate warm feelings. Furthermore, if we are "in touch" with our own emotions, we develop empathy for other human beings. Even if we don't like a person, we know he feels pain when he gets a splinter and pleasure when he takes a bath.

Establishing strong attachments can be very difficult for the child with a tactile disorder. The overresponsive child may withdraw from ordinary affection, while the underresponsive child may disregard it.

Feeling empathy can also be hard. The overresponsive child feels pain or discomfort where others do not; the underresponsive child feels no pain or discomfort where others do. He cannot relate well to another person's feelings.

HOW THE TACTILE SENSE
AFFECTS A CHILD'S EMOTIONAL SECURITY

A Typical Child	*A Child with Tactile Dysfunction*
At nine, Mike takes pleasure in going away to Boy Scout camp. He is comfortable in novel settings and likes making new friends. One night the scouts play a creative thinking game: "What Would You Need on a Desert Isle?" Mike suggests a bucket to catch rainwater, a sleeping bag, and binoculars—familiar objects that he has handled—as well as someone to talk to. Mike's well-regulated tactile sense gives him emotional security.	James, nine, is unhappy at camp. He misses his mother. He depends on her totally and exclusively for emotional support and always wants her nearby. Forming attachments to others is hard because everyone else seems unreliable. When the scouts play the Desert Isle game, he has no suggestions; all he can think is that he hates the idea of being deserted, hates being a Boy Scout, and hates being away from home.

The child may have difficulty experiencing pleasure, enthusiasm, and joy in his relationships because of his responses to touch. While he needs even more love than others, he invites less. His insecurity in the world puts his emotional well being at risk, as a child and as an adult.

Indeed, many adult relationships flounder when one partner's tactile disorder interferes with emotional intimacy. Too little touching makes the other person feel rejected; too much makes the other feel disrespected.

Tactile disorder also limits a child's imagination. Fantasy and make-believe may be beyond his scope, and the differences between real and pretend may be vague. He may be a rigid, inflexible thinker.

Social Skills

A well-regulated tactile sense is fundamental for getting along well with others. Building on the primary mother-child bond, we begin to reach out to others, gladly and comfortably touching and being touched. When we enjoy being near people, we learn how to play, one of the unique characteristics of being human. Thus, it becomes possible to develop meaningful human relationships.

When the child responds to physical contact in ways that are incomprehensible to most people, he may turn them away. The sensory disregarder who doesn't notice touch will have difficulty in social situations, as will the sensory craver or "bad boy" who tackles others because he seeks deep-touch pressure, and the sensory jumbler, slumper, or fumbler who cannot use touch messages effectively.

The sensory avoider or "sissy" who withdraws from touch has particular problems with socialization. Standoffish behavior sends signals that he is unfriendly and prefers to be left alone. Seeming to reject others, he is rejected in turn. He has difficulty dealing with the give-and-take, rough-and-tumble world of "playground politics."

Children with tactile defensiveness frequently mature into adults who are "cool characters." They may be cautious, controlled,

HOW THE TACTILE SENSE
AFFECTS A CHILD'S SOCIAL SKILLS

A Typical Child	*A Child with Tactile Dysfunction*
Standing in line to go to the lunch-room, Jake, eight, playfully bumps into Lewis. Lewis bumps him back. Laughing, they collide a few more times until all the third-graders are lined up and ready to go. When the teacher turns her attention to them and raises her eyebrow, the boys regain control and walk peacefully down the hall. Jake's positive reaction to tactile sensations is the foundation of his good social skills.	Curtis, eight, always tries to be last in line so no one is behind him. But today, Eli brings up the rear and grazes him as they go down the hall. Overresponding, Curtis punches Eli. Eli punches back. The boys begin to argue, and the teacher pulls them apart. Curtis complains, "Eli started it. It's his fault." Eli says, "I touched him accidentally! He's such a baby." Relating to his peers is hard because Curtis is uneasy when they get near.

and often inflexible people. They may seem distrustful or judgmental. Their behavior may be considered "touchy"—a funny word for people who avoid touch! Of course, they can develop social relationships with a select group, but the relationships are often built on shared interests that do not involve physical interaction.

CHARACTERISTICS OF
TACTILE DYSFUNCTION

The following checklists will help you gauge whether your child has tactile dysfunction. As you check recognizable characteristics, you will begin to see emerging patterns that help to explain your child's out-of-sync behavior. Not all characteristics will apply, but many checked boxes suggest that SPD affects your child.

The sensory avoider with **overresponsivity (tactile defensive-ness)** has difficulties with passive touch (being touched). He may:

☐ Respond negatively and emotionally to light-touch sensations, exhibiting anxiety, hostility, or aggression. He may withdraw from light touch, scratching or rubbing the place that has been touched. As an infant, he may have rejected cuddling as a source of pleasure or calming.

☐ Respond negatively and emotionally to the *possibility* of light touch. He may appear irritable or fearful when others are close, as when lining up.

☐ Respond negatively and emotionally when approached from the rear, or when touch is out of his field of vision, such as when someone's foot grazes his under a blanket or table.

☐ Show fight-or-flight response when touched on the face, such as having his face washed.

☐ Respond negatively when hairs on his body (arms, legs, neck, face, back, etc.) are displaced and "rubbed the wrong way." A high wind or even a breeze can raise his hairs, literally "ruffling his feathers."

☐ Show fight-or-flight response to hair displacement, such as having his hair brushed, or receiving a haircut, shampoo, or pat on the head.

☐ Become upset in weather with rain, wind, or gnats.

☐ Be excessively ticklish.

☐ Overrespond to physically painful experiences, making a "big deal" over a minor scrape or a splinter. The child may remember and talk about such experiences for days. He may be a hypochondriac.

☐ Respond similarly to dissimilar touch sensations. A raindrop on his skin may cause as adverse a response as a thorn.

☐ Strongly resist being touched by a barber, dentist, nurse, or pediatrician.

☐ Exhibit behavior that seems stubborn, rigid, inflexible, willful, verbally or physically pushy, or otherwise "difficult" for no apparent reason, when it is actually an aversive response to tactile stimuli.

☐ Rebuff friendly or affectionate pats and caresses, especially if the person touching is not a parent or familiar person. The child may reject touch altogether from anyone except his mother (or primary caregiver).

☐ Be distracted, inattentive, and fidgety when quiet concentration is expected.

☐ Prefer receiving a hug to a kiss. He may crave the deeptouch pressure of a hug, but try to rub off the irritating light touch of a kiss.

☐ Resist having his fingernails trimmed.

☐ Dislike surprises.

The same sensory avoider with **overresponsivity** also has difficulties with active touch. He may:

☐ Resist brushing his teeth.

☐ Be a picky eater, preferring certain textures such as crispy or mushy foods. The child may dislike foods with unpredictable lumps, such as tomato sauce or vegetable soup, as well as sticky foods like rice and cake icing.

☐ Refuse to eat hot or cold food.

☐ Avoid giving kisses.

☐ Resist baths, or insist that bath water be extremely hot or cold.

☐ Curl or protect hands to avoid touch sensations.

☐ Be unusually fastidious, hurrying to wash a tiny bit of dirt off his hands.

☐ Avoid walking barefoot on grass or sand, or wading in water.

☐ Walk on tiptoe to minimize contact with the ground.

☐ Fuss about clothing, such as stiff new clothes, rough textures, shirt collars, turtlenecks, belts, elasticized waists, hats, and scarves.

☐ Fuss about footwear, particularly sock seams. He may refuse to wear socks. He may complain about shoelaces. He may insist upon wearing beach sandals on cold, wet, winter days, or heavy boots on hot summer days.

☐ Prefer short sleeves and shorts and refuse to wear hats and mittens, even in winter, to avoid the sensation of clothes rubbing on his skin.

☐ Prefer long sleeves and pants and insist on wearing hats and mittens, even in summer, to avoid having his skin exposed.

☐ Avoid touching certain textures or surfaces, like some fabrics, blankets, rugs, or stuffed animals.

☐ Need to touch repeatedly certain surfaces and textures that provide soothing and comforting tactile experiences, such as a favorite blanket.

☐ Withdraw from art, science, music, and physical activities to avoid touch sensations.

☐ Avoid messy play, such as sand, finger paint, paste, glue, mud, and clay, perhaps becoming tearful at the idea.

☐ Stand still or move against the traffic in group activities such as obstacle courses or movement games, keeping constant visual tabs on others.

☐ Treat pets roughly, or avoid physical contact with pets.

☐ Arm himself at all times with a stick, toy, rope, or other handheld weapon.

☐ Rationalize verbally, in socially acceptable terms, why he avoids touch sensations, i.e., "My mother told me not to get my hands dirty," or "I'm allergic to mashed potatoes."

☐ Withdraw from a group and resist playing at other children's homes.

☐ Have trouble forming warm attachments with others. Experiencing difficulty in social situations, he may be a loner, with few close friends.

The sensory disregarder with **underresponsivity** may show atypical responses to passive and active touch. The child may:

☐ Not notice touch unless it is very intense.

☐ Be unaware of messiness on his face, especially around his mouth and nose, not noticing a crumby face or a runny nose.

☐ Be unaware of mussed hair or mulch or sand in hair.

☐ Not notice that clothes are in disarray, or that cuffs and socks are wet.

☐ Not notice heat, cold, or changes in temperature indoors or out, often keeping on a jacket even when sweating, or not reaching for a jacket even when shivering.

☐ Show little or no response to pain from scrapes, bruises, cuts, or shots, perhaps shrugging off a broken finger or collarbone.

☐ When barefoot, not complain about sharp gravel, hot sand, or stubbed toes.

☐ Not react to spicy, peppery, acidic, hot or "mouthburning" food—or, on the other hand, may crave this kind of food.

☐ Be oblivious to weather conditions with wind, rain, or gnats.

☐ Fail to realize that he has dropped something.

☐ Not move away when leaned on or crowded.

☐ Appear to lack "inner drive" to touch, handle and explore toys and materials that appeal to most other children.

☐ Require intense tactile stimulation to become engaged in the world around him, but not actively seek it.

☐ Hurt other children or pets during play, seemingly without remorse, but actually not comprehending the pain that others feel.

The sensory craver with **sensory seeking** needs extra touch stimuli, both passive and active. The child may:

☐ Ask for tickles or back rubs.

☐ Enjoy vibration or movement that provides strong sensory feedback.

☐ Need to touch and feel everything in sight, e.g., bumping and touching others and running hands over furniture and walls. The child has "gotta touch" items that other children understand are not to be touched.

☐ Rub certain textures over her arms and legs to get light-touch input.

☐ Rub or even bite his own skin excessively.

☐ Constantly twirl hair in fingers.

☐ Frequently remove socks and shoes.

☐ Seem compelled to touch or walk barefoot on certain surfaces and textures that other people find uncomfortable or painful.

☐ Seek certain messy experiences, often for long durations.

☐ Seek very hot or cool room temperature and bath water.

☐ Have high tolerance for sweltering summer or freezing winter weather.

☐ "Dive" into food, often cramming mouth with food.

☐ Prefer steaming hot, icy cold, extra-spicy, or excessively sweet foods.

☐ Use his mouth to investigate objects, even after the age of two. (The mouth provides more intense information than hands.)

☐ Show "in your face" behavior, getting very close to others and touching them, even if his touches are unwelcome.

The child having a problem with **tactile discrimination** may:

☐ Have poor body awareness and not know where his body parts are or how they relate to one another. He may seem "out of touch" with hands, feet, and other body parts, as if they are unfamiliar attachments.

☐ Be unable to identify which body parts have been touched without looking.

☐ Have trouble orienting his arms, hands, legs, and feet to get dressed.

☐ Be unable to identify familiar objects solely through touch, needing the additional help of vision, e.g., when reaching for objects in a pocket, box, or desk.

☐ Be unable to know the difference between similar items he is using, such as a crayon versus a marker.

☐ Be disheveled, with shoes on wrong feet, socks sagging, shoelaces untied, waistband twisted, and shirt untucked.

☐ Avoid initiating tactile experiences, such as picking up toys, materials, and tools that are attractive to others.

☐ Have trouble perceiving the physical properties of objects, such as their texture, shape, size, temperature, or density.

☐ Be fearful in the dark.

☐ Prefer standing to sitting, in order to ensure visual control of his surroundings.

☐ Act silly in the classroom, playing the role of "class clown."

☐ Have a limited imagination.

☐ Have a limited vocabulary because of inexperience with touch sensations.

The child with **dyspraxia** may:

☐ Have trouble conceiving of, organizing, and performing activities that involve a sequence of movements, such as cutting, pasting, coloring, assembling collage pieces or recipe ingredients, applying nail polish, and so forth. Novel experiences as well as familiar activities may be difficult.

☐ Have poor gross-motor control for running, climbing, and jumping.

☐ Have poor eye-hand coordination.

☐ Require visual cues to perform certain motor tasks that other children can do without looking, such as zipping, snapping, buttoning, and unbuttoning clothes.

☐ Put on gloves or socks in unusual ways.

☐ Have poor fine-motor control of his fingers for precise manual tasks, e.g., holding and using eating utensils and classroom tools, such as crayons, scissors, staplers, and hole punchers.

☐ Struggle with handwriting, drawing, completing work-sheets, and similar tasks.

☐ Have poor fine-motor control of his toes for walking barefoot or in flip-flops.

☐ Have poor fine-motor control of his mouth muscles for sucking, swallowing, chewing, and speaking.

☐ Be a messy eater.

☐ Have poor self-help skills and not be a "self-starter," requiring another person's help to get going.

Your child's primary problem may be with the tactile sense. He may also have difficulty with the internal vestibular and proprioceptive senses, as well as with the external visual and auditory senses.

Chapter Four

How to Tell if Your Child Has a Problem With The Vestibular Sense

Two First-Graders at the Amusement Park

Jason Green is in perpetual motion, but is not much of a conversationalist. He is a "high motor, low verbal" kid. When he began to talk at three, his few words included "choo, choo" and "toot, toot," for his passion is trains. Jason loves trains so much that his father calls him "our little locomotive."

Kevin Brown, Jason's best buddy, loves trains, too. Kevin behaves not like a train, however, but like a conductor. He is a "low motor, high verbal" child. His mother jokingly calls him "NATO," for "No Action, Talk Only."

When the boys play, Kevin bosses Jason around, and Jason cheerfully obeys. Once, Kevin proposed making a train by hitching together a little red wagon, a Big Wheel, and an old tricycle. Jason nodded agreement. All thumbs, the boys fumbled with rope and finally managed to connect the vehicles. Then Kevin instructed

Jason to push the train down his steep driveway so they could watch it plummet into the garage.

Instead of pushing the train, however, Jason clambered into the wagon. "Toot, toot!" he yelled as he plunged down the driveway. Kevin froze. He watched, helpless and horrified, as the train careened out of control.

Jason landed in a heap. He heaved himself up and said, "That was awesome! Totally fantastic! Want to try, Kevin?"

For once, Kevin was speechless.

Today is Jason's sixth birthday, and his parents are taking the boys to the amusement park. Jason loves the Ferris wheel, the merry-go-round, and especially the roller coaster. His idea of heaven is being twirled and tilted in the huge "Teacup." He never even gets dizzy.

Kevin is less enthusiastic. He has never found amusement parks amusing, because moving fast, high, and around in circles makes him tip over or fall, and the thought frightens him. He likes only the little train that slowly circles the park.

The first attraction the group approaches is the "Greased Toboggan." At the top of a slick ramp, riders sit in padded sacks and then slide down. Jason eagerly pulls on his father's sleeve to get his attention and permission.

Mr. Brown and Jason mount the stairs to the top. Jason ascends as fast as he can in his "marking time" fashion. He puts both feet on each step: right first, then left. In his haste, he stumbles twice.

Kevin lingers below with Mrs. Brown, watching. He doesn't want to slide; he wants to conduct. He raises his arms and shouts, "Go!" each time someone begins to descend. When he lifts his arms, his shoulders rise, too.

Mrs. Brown asks Kevin if he would like to get into a sack with Jason. She points out that lots of people are coming down together in the same sack.

"Oh, no, thank you very much," Kevin says. "You see, I can't slide down the ramp because I have to tell everyone when to go. I have to make sure that everyone is doing it just right."

Jason and Mr. Brown swoop to the bottom. "That was so awesome!" Jason says. "Now let's go to the roller coaster. That's the most fun of all."

Kevin says, "No, let's go to the train. That's entertaining, and it isn't dangerous for children."

Jason is disappointed but agrees to do whatever his friend wants.

Toot, toot! Chug, chug! Off they go.

Atypical Patterns of Behavior

Kevin and Jason approach movement experiences very differently. They both show atypical patterns of behavior.

Moving and being moved dismay Kevin. He is uncomfortable on slides and rides that move fast or spin around. He is afraid of heights and prefers to keep his feet on the ground. He relies on his precocious verbal skills to maintain control. Having sensory modulation dysfunction, and overresponsive to most vestibular sensations, Kevin is intolerant of movement and has gravitational insecurity.

In contrast, moving and being moved thrill Jason. Constantly and impulsively, he seeks fast-moving and spinning activities, but he does not get dizzy. Having the modulation disorder of sensory seeking, Jason craves movement, but his movements are disorganized.

In addition to modulation problems, both boys have sensory-based motor disorder. Kevin has dyspraxia, which interferes with carrying out his complex plan to make a train. On top of that, he has postural disorder, which makes it hard to isolate his movements to raise just one arm without raising the other arm and his shoulders to boot.

Jason, too, fumbles with the rope and stumbles up the stairs because of dyspraxia and poor bilateral coordination. Jason also has language problems. To communicate, he often uses gestures such as nodding his head or tugging on his father. He tends to be more talkative, however, after intense vestibular experiences such as sliding down the driveway and riding the Greased Toboggan.

On the next pages you will learn how the vestibular sense is supposed to function, followed by an explanation of the types of dysfunction that derail Kevin and Jason.

THE SMOOTHLY FUNCTIONING
VESTIBULAR SENSE

The vestibular system tells us about up and down and whether we are upright or not. It tells us where our heads and bodies are in relation to the earth's surface. It sends sensory messages about balance and movement from the neck, eyes, and body to the CNS for processing and then helps generate muscle tone so we can move smoothly and efficiently.

This sense tells us whether we are moving or standing still, and whether objects are moving or motionless in relation to our body. It also informs us what direction we are going in, and how fast we are going. This is extremely useful information should we need to make a fast getaway! Indeed, the fundamental functions of fight, flight, and foraging for food depend on accurate information from the vestibular system. Dr. Ayres writes that the "system has basic survival value at one of the most primitive levels, and such significance is reflected in its role in sensory integration."

The receptors for vestibular sensations are hair cells in the inner ear, which is like a "vestibule" for sensory messages to pass through. The inner-ear receptors work something like a carpenter's level. They register every movement we make and every change in head position—even the most subtle.

Some inner-ear structures receive information about where our head and body are in space when we are motionless, or move slowly, or tilt our head in any linear direction—forward, backward, or to the side. As an example of how this works, stand up in an ordinary biped, or two-footed, position. Now, close your eyes and tip your head way to the right. With your eyes closed, resume

113

your upright posture. Open your eyes. Are you upright again, where you want to be? Your vestibular system did its job.

Other structures in the inner ear receive information about the direction and speed of our head and body when we move rapidly in space, on the diagonal or in circles. Stand up and turn around in a circle or two. Do you feel a little dizzy? You should. Your vestibular system tells you instantly when you have had enough of this rotary stimulation. You will probably regain your balance in a moment.

What stimulates these inner ear receptors? Gravity!

According to Dr. Ayres, gravity is "the most constant and universal force in our lives." It rules every move we make.

Throughout evolution, we have been refining our responses to gravitational pull. Our ancient ancestors, the first fish, developed gravity receptors, on either side of their heads, for three purposes:

1) to keep upright,

2) to provide a sense of their own motions so they could move efficiently, and

3) to detect potentially threatening movements of other creatures through the vibrations of ripples in the water.

Millions of years later, we still have gravity receptors to serve the same purposes—except now vibrations come through air rather than water.

In addition to the inner ear, we humans also have outer ears as well as a cerebral cortex, which processes precise vestibular and auditory sensations. These sensations are the vibrations of movement and of sound.*

Nature designed our vestibular receptors to be extremely sensitive. *Indeed, our need to know where we are in relation to the*

---

* Vibrations stir up all kinds of responses. One day in my music class, I introduced a movement activity by beating a large drum. "Oooo," said a three-year-old girl, "I can feel that in my bones!" "Me, too," responded a little boy, "and I can even feel it in my penis!"

earth is more compelling than our need for food, for tactile comfort, or even for a mother-child bond.

In her book, *Sensory Integration and the Child*, Dr. Ayres explains:

> The vestibular system is the unifying system. It forms the basic relationship of a person to gravity and the physical world. All other types of sensation are processed in reference to this basic vestibular information. The activity in the vestibular system provides a "framework" for the other aspects of our experience. Vestibular input seems to "prime" the entire nervous system to function effectively. When the vestibular system does not function in a consistent and accurate way, the interpretation of other sensations will be inconsistent and inaccurate, and the nervous system will have trouble "getting started."

Whew! What a heavy load! Isn't it astonishing how something you may never have heard of before has such a profound and pervasive influence? As the background for all other senses, the vestibular system gives us a sense of where we stand in the world.

This system, like other sensory systems, has a defensive component. When an infant feels herself falling, she responds to this vestibular sensation as if saying, "Uh, oh!" She extends her arms and legs, groping for something to grab. Her whole body responds in this automatic, self-protective reflex.

As a child grows, her brain integrates reflexive responses in a process called reflex maturation. She learns to discriminate vestibular sensations. She seems to say, "Aha! I'm learning to sense what direction I'm going in and whether my movement is fast or slow."

Now, when movement sensations help her perceive that she is off center, she learns how to regain her balance. She learns to "stand on her own two feet," in an upright position, against the pull of gravity. She learns to differentiate her body movements so she can function with an economy of motion.

She can also discriminate among the sounds vibrating in her inner ear, and she learns to listen. She can coordinate her own body movements with visual sensations, and she learns to discriminate what she sees.

She learns to enjoy all kinds of movement. One kind is linear movement—back-and-forth, side-to-side, or up-and-down. Slow and low linear movement, which does not challenge gravity, is usually soothing. Parents have known since time immemorial that they can comfort a baby in a rocking chair, in a cradle, or with gentle bounces. In fact, many children (and adults) rock themselves when they are upset, as a kind of tranquilizing self-therapy.

Another kind of movement is rotary—moving around and around. Examples of rotary movement include spinning oneself on a tight axis, (e.g., planting one foot on the ground and turning rapidly), riding on a merry-go-round, or swinging high on a long-roped swing. Most children enjoy twirling on a tire swing—even to the point of getting dizzy. Rotary movement stimulates the vestibular system. Usually, it feels good, and that's why it is so much fun!

THE OUT-OF-SYNC VESTIBULAR SENSE

Vestibular dysfunction is the inefficient processing in the brain of sensations received through the inner ear. The child with a vestibular problem has difficulty processing information about gravity, balance, and movement through space.

The child may not develop the postural responses needed to keep upright. She may never have crawled or crept and may be late learning to walk. She may sprawl on the floor, slump when she sits, and lean her head on her hands when she is at the table.

As she grows, she may be awkward and uncoordinated at playground games. She may fall often and easily, tripping on air when she moves, bumping into furniture, and losing her balance when someone moves her slightly off center.

As eye movements are influenced by the vestibular system,

she may have visual problems. She may have inadequate gaze stability and be unable to focus on moving objects or on objects that stay still while she moves. At school, she may become confused when looking up at the board and down to her desk. Reading problems may arise if she hasn't developed brain functions imperative for coordinating left-to-right eye movements.

Vestibular dysfunction may also contribute to difficulty processing language—a great disadvantage in everyday life. The child who misperceives language may have problems learning to communicate, read, and write.

Many movements provide a calming effect. The out-of-sync child, however, can't always calm herself because her brain can't modulate vestibular messages. Difficulty moving smoothly interferes with her behavior, attention, self-esteem, and emotions. The child with an inefficient vestibular system may have modulation, discrimination and motor problems affecting her every move.

Sensory Modulation Disorders

VESTIBULAR OVERRESPONSIVITY—"OH, NO!"
Vigorous movement, or the possibility of being moved, causes the child with vestibular overresponsivity to respond negatively and emotionally, or to become overexcited.

This modulation disorder means that her brain can't regulate movement sensations. Her vestibular system is on overload. Particularly when her head or eyes move, her brain is bombarded with sensory stimuli that it can't organize. Two types of vestibular overresponsivity are intolerance to movement and gravitational insecurity.

INTOLERANCE TO MOVEMENT—"NO, DON'T!"
The child who is overresponsive to vestibular sensations may be intolerant of movement. Faulty processing causes aversive responses. "Oh, no, don't make me move! Moving quickly is too much for me."

HOW INTOLERANCE TO MOVEMENT
AFFECTS A CHILD'S BEHAVIOR

A Typical Child	A Child with Intolerance to Movement
Noah's favorite activities are movement and music. Today, the preschoolers play "Noncompetitive Musical Chairs." In this game, no chair is ever taken away. The object is to move around the chairs while the music plays and sit on any seat when the music stops. Everyone plays the whole time; no one is ever "out." When the music starts, Noah jumps up and circles the chairs with the other kids. When the music stops, he slithers into a chair. Once, he lands on another child's lap, but he looks around fast, sees an empty chair, and runs to it. Safe!	Sean, four, dislikes most music and movement activities. "Noncompetitive Musical Chairs" makes him especially uncomfortable. While the other children run freely around the circle, he inches along, clinging to the seats of the chairs. By the time he has circled the chairs twice, his forehead is sweaty, and his stomach is churning. The music finally stops, and Sean sits down with a sigh of relief. When the music resumes, he remains seated.

For her, linear movement is distressing, especially when rapid. Riding in a car—particularly in the back seat—often causes car sickness. She may avoid riding a bicycle, sliding and swinging at the playground, or just walking down the street.

Rotary movement can be even more distressing. She may become easily dizzy and nauseated on a tire swing. Even watching someone or something spinning can make her feel queasy. Moving in circles may make her head ache and stomach hurt.

If she avoids moving, she may lose the ability to keep up with others. She may become breathless and easily fatigued. Her motor planning skills and coordination may suffer, because she can't practice them with confidence.

GRAVITATIONAL INSECURITY—"I'M FALLING!"

Being connected to the earth is a primal need for survival. The vestibular system tells us where we are in relation to the ground. The trust that we are attached to the earth is called gravitational security.

Usually, a child has inner drive to experiment with gravity. Jumping, swinging, and somersaulting, she can relinquish her grip on earth for an instant, because she knows she will always return. With this basic sense of stability, she can develop emotional security.

The child with poor modulation may not enjoy this sense of stability. She feels vulnerable if her feet leave the ground. Lacking a basic sense of belonging to the earth, she has gravitational insecurity, or "G.I."

Gravitational insecurity is abnormal distress and anxiety in response to falling or the possibility of falling. *It is a primal fear.* It occurs when the child's brain overreacts to changes in gravity, even as subtle as standing up.

Movement for this child is not fun; it is scary. When her head moves, she responds, "I'm falling! I'm out of control!" She overreacts with a fight-or-flight response.

The "fight" response plays out as negative, defiant behavior, particularly when she is passively moved. She may resist being picked up, rocked, or pushed in the stroller. She may become angry and stubborn when someone suggests riding in the car or sledding down a hill.

The "flight" response plays out as extreme caution or avoidance of movement. She prefers keeping her head up and feet down, firmly planted. She may avoid playing "Ring Around the Rosy," riding a bicycle, sliding and swinging. She may be fearful of unstable surfaces, such as a sandy beach or a climbing net at the playground. She may avoid novel experiences, such as visiting a friend's house, because any place other than home is unpredictable.

The child with this terror tends to be inflexible and controlling. She often has social and emotional problems, because she is

HOW GRAVITATIONAL INSECURITY
AFFECTS A CHILD'S BEHAVIOR

A Typical Child	A Child with Gravitational Insecurity
With his class, Jack, nine, goes for a hike up a little mountain. At one point, a thick vine hangs down from a branch. Jack takes a turn swinging on the vine, screaming, "Tarzan!" Jack's efficient vestibular system permits him to enjoy exploring gravity as he swings and soars through the air.	The day his class goes hiking, Brad, nine, watches each step. He is grouchy, silent, and slow. He stands aloof while his classmates swing on a vine. When it's his turn, he takes the vine reluctantly. He can't move. The others cry, "Come on! What's your problem? It's fun!" Brad senses that if his feet leave the ground, he'll fall into the void. Saying, "I'm really not interested in this stupid game," he drops the vine and stalks away.

so worried about falling that she always feels vulnerable when around other people. The result is that she can't get organized for other tasks, such as playing and socializing.

VESTIBULAR UNDERRESPONSIVITY—"HO, HUM."
Another child may be underresponsive to movement experiences. She does not respond negatively; she simply does not seem to notice. As an infant, she may have been "such an easy baby," always ready to curl up in anyone's arms, always ready for a long, long nap. As she matures, she seems to lack inner drive to move actively. Although she requires extra movement to "get in gear," this child does not usually seek movement. Once started, however, she may have difficulty stopping.

Also, the child may be oblivious to the sensation of falling. She cannot respond efficiently with protective extension, i.e., extending a hand or a foot to catch herself. Many children with autism with this difficulty may have bruises because of frequent falls.

HOW VESTIBULAR UNDERRESPONSIVITY
AFFECTS A CHILD'S BEHAVIOR

A Typical Child	*A Child with Underresponsivity*
Jeff, thirteen, comes to the pool for aquatic therapy to strengthen his leg, which he broke while skiing last winter. On the concrete pool deck, he slips on a puddle and reacts immediately to catch himself, reaching for the wall so he doesn't fall and break the other leg. That's all he needs.	Cameron, a thirteen-year-old with autism, comes to the pool for aquatic therapy. Lumbering toward his recreational therapist, he slips on a puddle. Unaware of the sensation of falling, and slow to protect himself, he ricochets off the wall and collapses on the pool deck. The therapist rushes to his side and guides him into the soothing water before he has a meltdown.

VESTIBULAR SEEKING—"MORE!"

The child who craves vestibular sensations never seems to get enough of movements that are sufficiently satisfying for others. The child has an increased tolerance for movement. She seeks and enjoys a great deal of vigorous activity to satisfy her sensory needs.

To get vestibular sensations, the child may seek to resist gravity in unusual ways. For instance, she may assume upside-down positions, hang over the edge of her bed, or place her head down on the floor and pivot around it.

The child may frequently seek intense movement sensations, such as jumping from the top of the jungle gym, or running fast when a sedate pace would do. Climbing may be her passion; for the sensory craver, everything is a ladder.

She may crave linear movement and enjoy rocking or swinging for exceptionally long times. She may especially seek rotary movement, such as twirling in circles, shaking her head vigorously from side to side, or spinning on the playground merry-go-round or tire swing.

She may flit and dart from one activity to another, always

HOW SENSORY SEEKING
AFFECTS A CHILD'S BEHAVIOR

A Typical Child	A Child with Sensory Seeking
Justin, three, is at the swim center with his mother. He paddles in the kiddie pool, occasionally pausing to watch the big kids climb the ladder to the high diving board and jump into the water. When it is time to go home, he takes his mother's hand and says, "Let's go see that big ladder." He looks up, longingly. It's so high! So scary! Someday he'll be big and brave enough to climb it, but not yet.	Billy, three, is at the swim center with his mother. He starts to jump into the big pool, but she restrains him and guides him into the kiddie-pool enclosure. While she and the lifeguard discuss scheduling Billy's first swimming lesson, he escapes. He clambers up the high diving board. He teeters on the edge, ready to jump into the deep water. His mother notices his absence, springs up the ladder, and catches him just before he falls.

seeking a new thrill. Her attention span may be short, even for activities she enjoys. Although she may be constantly on the go, she may move without caution or good motor coordination.

HOW THE VESTIBULAR SENSE
AFFECTS EVERYDAY SKILLS

The vestibular sense gives us information necessary for many everyday skills:

- Gravitational security (see p. 120)
- Movement and balance
- Muscle tone
- Bilateral coordination
- Praxis (motor planning)
- Vision and hearing (see Chapters Six and Seven)
- Emotional security

Movement and Balance

Automatic, coordinated movement and balance are possible when the central nervous system connects vestibular sensations with other sensations. Movement and balance are sensory-based motor skills, not senses per se.

The vestibular system tells us which way is up, and that up is where we want to be. When we're upright, we're alert and in control. To keep upright, we make subconscious, physical adaptations, called postural background adjustments. These subtle adjustments allow us to stabilize our bodies, to correct and maintain our balance, and to move easily.

The child with vestibular dysfunction has problems with movement and balance. She moves too little or too much, with too much or too little caution. Her movements may be uncoordinated and awkward.

HOW MOVEMENT AND BALANCE
AFFECT A CHILD'S BEHAVIOR

A Typical Child	A Child with Vestibular Dysfunction
When Jeremy, ten, first got his skateboard, he fell frequently, but he has gradually learned to adjust his weight to keep his balance. He sets up obstacle courses in the street, with ramps and traffic cones, and invites his pals to try new tricks. When Joe collides with him and throws him off balance, Jeremy can usually land on his feet.	Joe, ten, can't quite get the hang of riding his skateboard, although he practices every day and works hard to master this skill. Yet he still crashes into Jeremy's ramps and traffic cones, and even into Jeremy. Usually Joe feels himself falling but can't stop himself, because his postural background adjustments are ineffective and he keeps losing his balance.

Muscle Tone

Muscle tone is the degree of tension normally present when our muscles are in a resting state. (Muscles never relax completely unless we are unconscious.) Muscle tone is a sensory-based motor skill and is a component of normal movement patterns. When we have good muscle tone, we usually take it for granted.

If you lead a normal life and exercise sometimes, you probably have adequate tone when you are resting. If you exercise regularly, you probably have firm tone. If you are a "couch potato," you probably have low tone. And, furthermore, if you are a couch potato—because the apple does not fall far from the tree—chances are that your child is a "potato chip."

The vestibular system, along with the proprioceptive system, strongly affects tone by regulating neurological information from the brain to the muscles, telling them exactly how much to contract, so that we can resist gravity to perform skilled tasks. Usually,

HOW MUSCLE TONE
AFFECTS A CHILD'S BEHAVIOR

A Typical Child	A Child with Vestibular Dysfunction
Scotty, four, pulls on his socks and his high-top sneakers. He doesn't yet know how to tie his shoes. He grips with his toes to keep the loose sneakers on his feet and thumps to his father for help. His father says, "You're growing so fast, soon you'll be able to tie your shoes all by yourself." Scotty says, "But I can make them twinkle. Want to see, Daddy?" He springs up, and when he lands, the heels of the sneakers light up.	Ted's father parks him on the bed and tries to push his limp feet into a pair of socks. "Can you help me, son?" he asks. "It seems as if I'm doing all the work here." Ted tries to cooperate, but his feet don't always do what he wants them to do. Finally, the socks are on. While his father wiggles Ted's feet into his sneakers, Ted sprawls backwards on the bed. "Can you help me, please?" asks his father. "Too tired," says Ted.

our muscle tone is neither too tight nor too loose; it is just right, so we don't have to use much effort to move our bodies or keep our-selves upright.

The child with vestibular dysfunction may have a "loose and floppy" body, or low tone. This is a postural disorder that inter-feres with her movement. Nothing is wrong structurally with her muscles, but her brain is not sending out sufficient messages to give them "oomph." Without that energizing oomph, the child's muscles lack the readiness or tension necessary to move with ease.

The sensory slumper may often lay her head on the table, or sprawl on the floor, or slouch in the chair. She may have difficulty turning knobs and pressing levers. She may handle objects loosely or with a very tight grasp in order to compensate for the underly-ing low muscle tone. She may tire easily, because resisting the pull of gravity requires a great deal of energy.

Bilateral Coordination

Bilateral (from the Latin for "both sides") coordination means that we can use both sides of the body to cooperate as a team. A well-regulated vestibular system helps us to integrate sensory messages from both sides of our body.

By the age of three or four, a child should be crossing the mid-line. For the child who avoids crossing the midline, coordinating both body sides may be difficult. When she paints at an easel, she may switch the brush from one hand to the other at the midway point separating her right and left sides. She may appear not to have established a hand preference, sometimes using her left and sometimes her right to eat, draw, write, or throw. It may also be hard to survey a scene or to track a moving object visually without stopping at the midline to blink and refocus.

The child with poor bilateral coordination may have trouble using both feet together to jump from a ledge, or both hands to-gether to catch a ball or play clapping games. She may have diffi-culty coordinating her hands to hold a paper while she cuts, or to stabilize the paper with one hand while she writes with the other.

Poor bilateral coordination, a sensory-based motor disorder, is often misinterpreted as a learning disability such as dyslexia. In fact, this difficulty can lead to learning or behavior problems, but it does not ordinarily mean that a child is lacking in intelligence or academic ability.

HOW BILATERAL COORDINATION
AFFECTS A CHILD'S BEHAVIOR

A Typical Child	A Child with Vestibular Dysfunction
Chelsea, eight, is making a Valentine. On a piece of red paper, she steadies a cardboard heart with her left hand and traces its outline with her right. She uses her right hand to cut out the heart and her left hand to hold and turn the paper. She makes four more Valentines during art period.	Celia, eight, wants to make a pink Valentine. She has trouble steadying the cardboard heart on the paper while she traces. Her outline is misshapen but will have to do. She picks up the paper in her right hand and the scissors in her left. No, that's not correct; she switches hands. She cuts awkwardly. Instead of rotating the paper with her left hand, she moves her right hand, holding the scissors, around the paper. Her Valentine isn't very good, but she hopes her mother will like it.

Visual and Auditory Processing

The vestibular system is intimately involved with vision and hearing. Please see the next chapters to learn more.

Praxis (Motor Planning)

Praxis, or motor planning, as you have seen, is the ability to conceptualize, organize, and realize a complex sequence of unfamiliar movements. When our nervous system integrates vestibular sensations with tactile and proprioceptive sensations, we have a good body scheme. When we have a good body scheme, we can motor plan. When we motor plan, we can accomplish what we set out to do.

HOW PRAXIS AFFECTS A CHILD'S BEHAVIOR

A Typical Child	A Child with Vestibular Dysfunction
Maddy, seven, likes learning new dances. Today the Brownies are mastering the Macarena, a dance that their Brownie leader, Mrs. Hopkins, learned in the 90s. In this dance, the girls move their arms and hands in a complicated sequence, turning them in the air and moving them to touch one body part after another. After completing the sequence, they shimmy, jump a quarter turn, and repeat the motions. The Macarena is much more challenging than the Looby Loo. Maddy loves this.	Libby likes being a Brownie, especially when the troop goes to museums and enacts stories, but she doesn't enjoy dancing. The Looby Loo was hard enough; now she must struggle with the Macarena. Moving her arms and hands is confusing and frustrating, because Libby has dyspraxia. Shimmying is difficult, so Libby just sways. Trying to jump a quarter turn, she goes in the wrong direction. Even when she stops to watch the other girls, it's hard to learn the sequence of movements. She wishes they could stick to familiar activities, instead of always tackling something new.

Adapting her behavior to learn a new skill may be very hard for the child with vestibular dysfunction. For instance, this sensory fumbler may be able to step into the bathtub, but have trouble stepping into the car. She may have learned how to roller skate, but have difficulty ice skating or rollerblading. If her central nervous system hasn't processed movement and balance sensations efficiently, then her brain can't remember how it feels to move in a certain way. Thus, she can't easily generalize a learned skill to plan and perform a new skill that is only slightly different.

Emotional Security

Emotional security is every child's birthright, but the child with vestibular dysfunction may not feel totally secure. With the inability to process where she stands and how she moves through space, she may be disorganized in many aspects of her young life.

The child may have low self-esteem. Aware that ordinary tasks are beyond her ability, she may often say, "I can't do that." She may not even try. If she is uncertain about her abilities, even the best-loved child in the world may feel unloved and unlovable.

HOW EMOTIONAL SECURITY
AFFECTS A CHILD'S BEHAVIOR

A Typical Child	*A Child with Vestibular Dysfunction*
Mark, four, gives Darius a huge, soft baseball and plastic bat for his birthday. After Darius unwraps the gift, Mark says, "Let's play!" A few children can wield the bat and whack the ball. Mark hits it over the fence. He claps his hands. "I knew I'd be good at this! Your turn, Darius." He offers the bat to his friend, but Darius frowns and turns away. When Mark's mother comes to pick him up, he says, "Darius didn't like the bat, Mommy, but that's okay. I had a good time at the party anyway."	Darius, four, opens Mark's present, but he doesn't want to play with the ball and bat. He knows he won't be any good. He watches the other children line up to swing the bat, but when Mark urges him to try, he turns away and says, "I can't." After the partygoers leave, he says to his mother, "Mark isn't my friend. He hates me." His eyes brim with tears, and he collapses in her arms. He whimpers, "Mommy, do you love me?"

CHARACTERISTICS OF VESTIBULAR
DYSFUNCTION

These checklists will help you gauge whether your child has vestibular dysfunction. As you check recognizable characteristics, you will begin to see emerging patterns that help to explain your child's out-of-sync behavior.

The overresponsive child who shows **intolerance for movement** may:

☐ Dislike playground activities, such as swinging, spinning, and sliding.

☐ Be cautious, slow moving, and sedentary, hesitating to take risks.

☐ Appear to be a sissy.

☐ Seem willful and uncooperative.

☐ Be very uncomfortable in elevators and on escalators, perhaps experiencing car or motion sickness.

☐ Demand continual physical support from a trusted adult.

The child with **gravitational insecurity** may:

☐ Have a great fear of falling, even where no real danger exists. This fear is experienced as primal terror.

☐ Be fearful of heights, even slightly raised surfaces. The child may avoid walking on a curb or jumping down from the bottom step.

☐ Become anxious when her feet leave the ground, feeling that even the smallest movement will throw her into outer space.

☐ Be fearful of climbing or descending stairs, and hold tightly to the banister.

☐ Feel threatened when her head is inverted, upside down or tilted, as when having her head shampooed over the sink.

☐ Be fearful when someone moves her, as when a teacher slides her chair closer to the table.

☐ For self-protection, try to manipulate her environment and other people.

☐ Have poor proprioception and poor visual discrimination.

The sensory disregarder with **underresponsiveness** to vestibular sensations may:

☐ Not notice or object to being moved.

☐ Seem to lack inner drive to move actively.

☐ Once started, swing for a lengthy time without getting dizzy.

☐ Not notice sensation of falling and may not respond efficiently to protect himself by extending his hands or a foot to catch himself.

The sensory-seeking child with **increased tolerance for movement** may:

☐ Need to keep moving, as much as possible, in order to function. The child may have trouble sitting still or staying in a seat.

☐ Repeatedly, vigorously shake her head, rock back and forth, and jump up and down.

☐ Crave intense movement experiences, such as bouncing on furniture, using a rocking chair, turning in a swivel chair, assuming upside-down positions, or placing her head on the floor and pivoting around it.

☐ Be a "thrill seeker," enjoying fast-moving or spinning playground equipment, or seeking the fast and "scary" rides at an amusement park.

☐ Not get dizzy, even after twirling or spinning rapidly for a lengthy amount of time.

☐ Enjoy swinging very high and/or for long periods of time.

☐ Like seesaws, teeter-totters, or trampolines more than other children.

The sensory slumper with sensory-based postural disorder affecting **movement of the head, balance, muscle tone, and bilateral coordination** may:

☐ Lose her balance unless both feet are firmly planted, as when stretching on tiptoes, jumping, or standing on both feet when her eyes are closed.

☐ Easily lose her balance when out of a biped (two-footed) position, as when climbing stairs, riding a bicycle, hopping, or standing on one foot.

☐ Move in an uncoordinated, awkward way.

☐ Be fidgety and clumsy.

☐ Have a loose and floppy body.

☐ Feel limp (like a wet noodle) when you lift her, move her limbs to help her get dressed, or try to help her balance on a teeter-totter or balance beam.

☐ Tend to slump or sprawl in a chair or over a table, prefer to lie down rather than sit upright, and constantly lean her head on a hand or arm.

☐ Find it hard to hold up her head, arms, and legs simultaneously when lying on her stomach.

☐ Sit on the floor with her legs in a "W," i.e., with her knees bent and her feet extended out to the sides, to stabilize her body.

☐ Have difficulty turning doorknobs or handles that require pressure, and have a loose grasp on "tools" such as pencils, scissors, or spoons.

☐ Have a tight, tense grasp on objects (to compensate for looseness).

☐ Have problems with digestion and elimination, such as frequent constipation or poor bladder control.

☐ Fatigue easily during physical activities or family outings.

☐ Be unable to catch herself from falling.

☐ Not have crawled or crept as a baby.

☐ Have poor body awareness.

☐ Have poor gross-motor skills and frequently stumble and trip, or be clumsy at sports and active games. She may seem to have "two left feet."

☐ Have poor fine-motor skills and difficulty using "tools" such as eating utensils, crayons, pencils, and combs.

☐ Have difficulty making both feet or both hands work together, such as when jumping up and down or throwing and catching a ball.

☐ Have difficulty using one foot or hand to assist the other during tasks such as standing on one foot to kick a ball, or holding the paper steady when writing or cutting.

☐ Have trouble using both hands in a smooth, alternating manner, as when striking rhythm instruments together to keep a musical beat.

☐ Not have an established hand preference by the age of four or five. The child may use either hand for coloring and writing, or may switch the crayon or pencil from one hand to the other.

☐ Avoid crossing the midline. The child may switch the brush from hand to hand while painting a horizontal line, or may have trouble tapping a hand on her opposite shoulder in games like "Simon Says."

☐ Have a hard time with organization and structured activities.

The sensory fumbler with **dyspraxia (poor motor planning)** may:

☐ Have difficulty conceptualizing, organizing, and carrying out a sequence of unfamiliar movements.

☐ Be unable to generalize what she has already learned in order to accomplish a new task.

The child who is **emotionally insecure** may:

☐ Get easily frustrated and give up quickly.

☐ Be reluctant to try new activities.

☐ Have a low tolerance for potentially stressful situations.

☐ Have low self-esteem.

☐ Be irritable in others' company, and avoid or withdraw from people.

☐ Have difficulty making friends and relating to peers.

Vestibular dysfunction may be your child's primary disorder, while the tactile sense (Chapter Three) and the proprioceptive sense (Chapter Five) may cause problems, too. Difficulties with visual and auditory processing are discussed in Chapters Six and Seven.

How to Tell if Your Child Has a Problem with the Proprioceptive Sense

One Nine-Year-Old at the Swimming Pool

Tony has tried to play team sports, but it's hard for him to get his body to work in a coordinated way. He hates it when other kids, including his siblings, say mean things like "You sure have a lousy sense of timing," or "Nobody picks you for a team because you don't help."

Knowing how Tony longs to participate in a sport, his mother persuades him to join the beginners' swim team at the neighborhood pool. After shopping for goggles, a team suit, and a new athletic bag, Tony begins to think that swimming might be okay. At least it doesn't involve hitting balls.

The first day of practice, Tony inches into the locker room. The other boys dart in and out, joking and laughing, while Tony struggles to change his clothes. He watches every move carefully, especially when he ties the waistband string of his swimsuit. He wants to be sure that his suit is on right, so nobody will laugh at him.

He goes out to the concrete pool deck and heads for the coach. He walks awkwardly, thudding his heels. He's watching his feet, not where he's going. He collides with a chair, which clatters across the concrete.

The coach glances up and beckons. He calls, "Come on! Get your goggles on! Dive in! Let's go!"

Getting the goggles on is tricky because Tony cannot see what he is doing. By the time he adjusts them, the other kids have dived in and begun swimming toward the far end of the pool.

Tony doesn't know how to dive, so getting into the pool is another problem. He goes to the ladder and faces the water. With his arms awkwardly stretched behind him as he clings to the railings, he tries to descend. Then he remembers to face the ladder, not the water. He turns around, gropes for the rungs with his feet, and backs slowly into the pool.

Tony begins to swim. He had swimming lessons, so he knows the basics. However, the pattern of his strokes is uneven. He stretches his right arm nicely but bends his left elbow too much, so he swims with a "limp." The result is that he keeps veering to the left and bumping into the rope.

Another problem is breathing. He concentrates hard: right arm, left arm, breathe, right, left, breathe—but he gets the sequence mixed up. When he breathes, his arms stop moving, and he feels as if he is about to sink.

When he gets to the end of the pool, Tony is exhausted. The other kids are already swimming back to the other end. He's always the last one. He thinks maybe swimming is not such a good idea after all.

Atypical Pattern of Behavior

Tony is out of sync with his body and moves in an atypical pattern. He strikes his heels on the pool deck to get additional information to his muscles and joints. His awkward gait makes him look like a robot.

Tony has poor body awareness: He cannot perceive how his

individual body parts move, or where they are in space. He relies on vision to figure out how to make his body move. Changing into his swimsuit takes a long time because he must watch his hands. Positioning his goggles over his eyes is hard because he can't see what he's doing.

Another challenge is orienting his body to get into the pool. First, Tony has trouble aligning his body properly on the ladder. Then, when he remembers to turn toward the ladder and to back into the water, he labors to find secure footing on the rungs.

In the pool, Tony's swimming is irregular. His strokes are erratic because matching his arm movements is difficult.

Tony works hard to swim; he likes the water and wants to be successful. He is easily frustrated, however, and decides that swimming isn't his thing. Uncoordinated and unaware of his body, Tony has proprioceptive dysfunction, and, as is common, dyspraxia and some vestibular dysfunction as well.

On the next pages you will find an explanation of how the proprioceptive sense is supposed to function, followed by an explanation of the types of dysfunction that sink Tony.

THE SMOOTHLY FUNCTIONING
PROPRIOCEPTIVE SENSE

Proprioception tells us about our own movement and body position. ("Proprio" means "one's own" in Latin.) Like "internal eyes," proprioception informs us:

- Where our body or body parts are in space,
- How our body parts relate to one another,
- How much and how quickly our muscles are stretching,
- How fast our body is moving through space,
- How our timing is, and
- How much force our muscles put forth.

This kind of information is fundamental for every move we make. Our reflexes, automatic responses and planned action (praxis) depend on it. The self-awareness that proprioception grants lets us do our job, whether we are a master violinist, downhill skier, or salad chef . . . or an apprentice tricycle rider, cookie snitcher, or book-report writer.

Proprioception is both subconscious, such as when we automatically hold our bodies upright on a chair, and conscious, such as when we uncross our legs before arising from the chair. Sometimes teachers and therapists use the term "kinesthesia" to describe the conscious awareness of joint position we use in learning, and it means the same thing.

Proprioception is the "position sense" or the "muscle sense." Receptors are mostly in the muscles and skin, and also in the joints, ligaments, tendons, and connective tissue. The stimulus for these receptors is stretch. When muscles or skin stretch or contract, and body parts bend and straighten, messages inform the central nervous system (CNS) about where and how the movement occurs.

We get the most and best proprioception when we actively stretch and tighten our muscles in resistive motions, against the pull of gravity—say, when we do a push-up or heavy work, such as hoisting a loaded laundry basket. When we are passively moved— say, when a salesclerk lifts our foot to insert it into a shoe—we get modest proprioception.

Even when we are motionless, we receive proprioceptive messages without being consciously aware of them. For instance, if you are seated right now and close your eyes, you are relying on proprioception, not vision, to tell you that you are resting in a chair. Are your feet on a stool? Do your hands hold this book? Proprioception gives you this information without the need to look at your feet and hands.

Muscle sensations that come through the proprioceptive system are closely connected to both the tactile and the vestibular systems. Proprioception helps integrate touch and movement sensations. Because they are so interrelated, professionals sometimes speak of "tactile-proprioceptive" or "vestibular-proprioceptive" processing.

Tactile-proprioceptive (or "somatosensory") discrimination refers to the simultaneous sensations of touch and of body position. This skill is necessary for such ordinary tasks as judging the weight of a glass of milk, or holding a pencil efficiently in order to write.

Vestibular-proprioceptive discrimination refers to the simultaneous sensations of head and body position when the child actively moves. This is needed for throwing and catching a ball, or climbing stairs.

What do we need proprioception for? The functions of proprioception are to increase body awareness and to govern motor control and motor planning. Proprioception contributes to visual discrimination; the more we move, the better we make sense of what we see. It helps us with body expression, the ability to sequence our motions and move our body parts efficiently and economically. It allows us to walk smoothly, to run quickly, to carry a suitcase, to sit, to stand, to stretch, and to lie down. It gives us emotional security, for when we can trust our bodies, we feel safe and secure.

Another very important function is to help modulate our arousal level. It brings you up when you're way down, and down when you're way up. Proprioceptive experiences calm and organize us, bringing us back to center when we have been under- or overstimulated in *any* of the other senses. For instance, the proprioceptive input from pushing against a wall, pulling on rubber tubing, or hanging from a trapeze bar can arouse a person who has been sitting all day. The very same input can calm a person who suffers from sensory overload in a busy classroom.

Furthermore, the calm and organization that proprioceptive input instills may last a couple of hours, and the person can tap into it to help himself function. Teachers, parents, and therapists who understand this phenomenon know that the best way to get children to settle down for a story or to do their homework is by first providing abundant opportunities for stretching and resistive activities.

An additional function of proprioception is the discrimination of movement in time and space. An example is tying shoelaces, which requires good proprioception of the muscles in the fingers, coordinated with good visual and tactile discrimination. To know when to let go of one end of the shoelace, and how big to make a loop, and where to stick that loop, we need praxis, praxis, praxis. As an adult, you may be able to tie laces in the dark and in your sleep; imagine trying to do it without proprioception.

THE OUT-OF-SYNC
PROPRIOCEPTIVE SENSE

Proprioceptive dysfunction is the inefficient processing of sensations perceived through the muscles and skin, as well as the joints. Proprioceptive dysfunction is almost always accompanied by problems with the tactile and/or vestibular systems. Whereas it is common for a child to have only a tactile problem or only a vestibular problem, it is less likely for a child to have only a proprioceptive problem.

The child with poor proprioception has difficulty interpreting sensations about the position and movement of his body parts. His CNS is inefficient at modulating these ordinarily subconscious sensations. Whether underresponsive or sensory seeking, he may be unable to use this information for adaptive behavior. He may show confusion when walking down the street, getting in and out of the bathtub, or crossing the playground. He may tackle everything and everybody.

Discriminating where his body parts are and the rate and speed of his movements is a problem. Because he cannot monitor his gross-motor and fine-motor muscles, motor control and praxis are challenging. He may be clumsy and easily frustrated. Other people perceive him to be a "klutz."

Manipulating objects may be difficult. He may exert too much or too little pressure on objects, struggling to turn doorknobs and regularly breaking toys and pencil points. He may spill the milk every time. The child may have a poor grip on heavy objects, such as buckets of water, or on lightweight objects, such as forks and combs. He may also have trouble lifting and holding on to objects of different weights.

Because of poor body awareness, the child needs to use his eyes to see what his body is doing. Ordinary tasks, such as orienting his body to get dressed, zipping a jacket, buttoning a shirt, or getting out of bed in the dark, become very difficult without the aid of vision. Unless the child can watch every move, he may be unable to match a movement of one side of his body with a similar movement on the other side.

The child may be fearful when moving in space because he lacks postural stability. Because each new movement and each new position throws him off guard, he is emotionally insecure.

The child with an inefficient proprioceptive system may have modulation, discrimination, and motor problems affecting his every move.

Sensory Modulation Disorders

PROPRIOCEPTIVE OVERRESPONSIVITY—"OH, NO!"
The child who is overresponsive to proprioception may avoid stretching and contracting his muscles. He may have poor body awareness and be rigid, tense, and uncoordinated. He lacks "internal eyes" to help him "see" what his body parts are doing.

He may shun playground activities with a lot of sensory input, such as jumping, hopping, running, bouncing, crawling, and rolling. He may resist getting into unusual positions, such as moving like animals, wriggling between the bars of a climber, or doing calisthenics in P.E. class. Not only active movement, but also passive movement may cause high anxiety when he is tightly hugged or when someone moves his arms and legs.

HOW OVERRESPONSIVITY
AFFECTS A CHILD'S BEHAVIOR

A Typical Child	*A Child with Overresponsivity*
Dominique, thirteen, at a Japanese restaurant for the first time, tries octopus and squid. The texture is rubbery. As she chews and chews, she compares the sensation to other foods she has had before. This is not like other seafood, she decides, but more like licorice or gum.	At the Japanese restaurant, Tia, thirteen, wants to be a good sport, so she tries a tiny piece of squid. It feels like chewing rubber, which is not OK. She removes the morsel from her mouth and hides it in her napkin. Then she concentrates on the rice.

Overresponsivity may also cause the child to be a picky eater. The reason is that certain food textures require forceful, coordinated chewing, and his mouth muscles are not getting the necessary sensory information.

PROPRIOCEPTIVE UNDERRESPONSIVITY—
"HO, HUM."

The child who is underresponsive to proprioception seems to lack the inner drive to move and play. He often has poor somatosensory (tactile-proprioceptive) discrimination, as well as postural problems and dyspraxia. This child tends to "fix," e.g., jam his elbow to his ribs for more input when trying to write, to compensate for postural instability.

Like the child with overresponsivity, he lacks "internal eyes," has poor body awareness, and is unusually clumsy with toys and materials. Unlike the sensory avoider, however, the sensory disregarder may not notice that he has been sitting for a long time in an uncomfortable position. The sensation of pins and needles may not bother him. He may be unable to orient his body to get dressed and may not care whether someone moves his arms and legs when the dressing job must be done. "Ho, hum."

HOW UNDERRESPONSIVITY AFFECTS
A CHILD'S BEHAVIOR

A Typical Child	A Child with Underresponsivity
Eden, twelve, has been sitting on the couch for an hour, engrossed in a Harry Potter book. She feels stiff and needs to move. She stands up, laces her hands together and pushes them out in front of her chest, overhead, from side to side, and behind her head. She repeats the stretching sequence, this time with her palms facing outward. Ahh, her body feels much better.	Destiny, twelve, has been in one position all day, deep into *Lord of the Rings*. Her mother calls. Destiny arises stiffly and stumbles to the kitchen to help prepare dinner. Because she tends to break dishes and cut herself while slicing vegetables, her mother gives her jobs that provide sensory input without doing any damage. Destiny scrubs potatoes, mixes meatloaf ingredients, squeezes lemons, tosses the salad, and takes out the garbage. Now she feels more alert.

Parents and teachers may notice that the sensory disregarder becomes more alert and organized after heavy work activity. Of course, this child needs someone to get him started. Chores around the house and classroom help, as does sensory integration intervention that provides plenty of proprioceptive feedback to increase arousal level.

PROPRIOCEPTIVE SEEKING—"MORE!"

The sensory seeking child is a "bumper and crasher." He craves active movement, pushing, pulling, making "crash landings" by throwing himself to the ground, and lunging into walls, tables, and people. He craves passive input to muscles and joints, as well, such as strong bear hugs, and being pressed, squeezed, or pummeled while roughhousing.

Always seeking more proprioceptive input, the sensory craver may bite, kick, hit, and behave in a seemingly aggressive manner. Some sensory cravers will engage in self-stimulation, such as biting their own skin or banging their head against the crib or wall. These children benefit from sensory integration treatment with ample opportunities for vigorous proprioceptive input to decrease their high arousal.

HOW PROPRIOCEPTIVE SEEKING
AFFECTS A CHILD'S BEHAVIOR

A Typical Child	*A Child with Sensory Seeking*
Before doing errands, Aaron, five, and his father go to the playground. Aaron can pump on the swing and he likes to move forward and back under his own steam. Now, they are at the grocery store. Aaron helps with the grocery cart. Pushing it forward and pulling it back feels good in his arms, abdomen, and back. On one forward thrust the cart accidentally bumps into the apple bin and a few apples go flying—one right into the cart! Aaron's father raises an eyebrow. Aaron restrains himself and just pushes and pulls the cart a little bit.	Chase, five, and his mother are in the fresh produce aisle. She is in a hurry and he is cranky. He refuses to ride in the kiddie seat, so she lets him push the grocery cart. He pushes and pulls the cart, to and fro, and then leans forward and strikes his head repeatedly on the handlebar. He can't see where he's going and crashes into a barrel of peanuts. That felt good! Before his mother can stop him, Chase deliberately shoves the cart into a display of cantaloupes. Next time they do errands together, Chase's mother will be sure that he has time to run and play beforehand.

How the Proprioceptive Sense Affects Everyday Skills

Proprioception works closely with the tactile and vestibular systems, so some functions overlap. These functions include:

- Body awareness
- Motor control
- Grading of movement

- Postural stability
- Praxis (Motor planning)
- Emotional security

Body Awareness

Efficient proprioception provides information about body awareness. The child with poor proprioception may be unaware of his body position and body parts.

HOW BODY AWARENESS AFFECTS A CHILD'S BEHAVIOR

A Typical Child	A Child with Proprioceptive Dysfunction
To settle the children down before reading a story, the teacher of Jonathan's preschool class leads a stretching exercise. She says, "Close your eyes and stretch one arm way up toward the ceiling. Bring it down and now stretch the other arm, way up high." Jonathan, three, follows her directions without difficulty.	Kenny, three, keeps his eyes open during the stretching exercise. He looks at his right arm to make sure it is moving. When the teacher says to stretch the other arm, Kenny peeks at Jonathan to see what he is doing. Attempting to imitate Jonathan, he gets confused. He raises his right arm again, rather than his left.

Motor Control

Proprioception provides information necessary to coordinate basic gross-motor and fine-motor movements. The child with poor proprioception has difficulty controlling large-motor movements, such as getting from one position into another, and fine-motor movements, such as grasping objects.

HOW MOTOR CONTROL
AFFECTS A CHILD'S BEHAVIOR

A Typical Child	*A Child with Proprioceptive Dysfunction*
Gary, eleven, rounds up some kids for a game of Horse. One by one, each child chooses a spot, and everyone takes a turn to stand there and shoot the basketball into the hoop. With every missed basket, a player gets a letter—H, O, R, S, and E. Gary has good motor control and rarely accumulates all the letters to spell Horse, which would put him out of the game.	Jasper, eleven, tries to play Horse on the basketball court. It is his turn and he takes the ball. His motor control is out of sync because discriminating sensations of body position and muscle movement is hard. He tries to catapult the ball into the hoop, but his muscles are too weak. He misses and gets an H. Then he gets an O, an R, an S, and an E. He's out.

Grading of Movement

Proprioception helps us grade our movements. Grading of movement means that we sense how much pressure to exert as we flex and extend our muscles. We can judge what the quantity and quality of muscle movement should be, and how forcefully we should move. Thus, we can gauge the amount of effort necessary to pick up a fluffy dust ball, lift a heavy carton, or yank open a stubborn drawer.

Suppose you're at a picnic, and you set down your lemonade on the table beside someone else's empty cup. Later, you return for another refreshing sip but pick up the other person's cup. You sense immediately that this cup is not yours, because it doesn't feel full. And how do you know? Proprioception tells you so!

Because the child with dysfunction does not receive efficient messages from his muscles and joints, he has difficulty grading his movements to adapt to changing demands.

HOW GRADING OF MOVEMENT AFFECTS A CHILD'S BEHAVIOR

A Typical Child	A Child with Proprioceptive Dysfunction
Janie, seven, is going to help paint the bike shed at camp. She carries a brush in one hand and a paint bucket in the other. Walking to the shed, she adjusts her body to keep upright despite carrying different weights.	Ruth, seven, holds a brush tightly in one hand so she won't drop it. Her counselor gives her a bucket of paint. As Ruth can't perceive how heavy it is, she can't tighten her muscles to stand upright. She leans way over to one side as she lugs the bucket.

Postural Stability

Proprioception gives us the subconscious awareness of our body that helps us stabilize ourselves when we sit, stand, and move. The child with dysfunction lacks the stability to make fundamental postural adjustments for these everyday skills.

HOW POSTURAL STABILITY
AFFECTS A CHILD'S BEHAVIOR

A Typical Child	A Child with Proprioceptive Dysfunction
Larry, ten, pulls in his chair and surveys the dinner table. Yippee, corn on the cob! He eats, with his elbows on the table. His mother says, "Manners, please," and he straightens up.	Adam, ten, arranges himself on the chair: one foot tucked under his body and the other on the floor for stability. He knows his mother disapproves of elbows on the table, but he can't help it when he eats corn.

Praxis (Motor Planning)

Praxis depends on accurate modulation and discrimination of proprioceptive messages. Planning and sequencing motor action is a challenge for people with dyspraxia, especially if they have underresponsivity.

HOW PRAXIS (MOTOR PLANNING)
AFFECTS A CHILD'S BEHAVIOR

A Typical Child	A Child with Dyspraxia
Todd, six, is practicing a marching routine in preparation for Field Day. "*Hup*, two, three, four, *hup*, two, three, four," he chants as he smartly brings up his knees. When the P.E. teacher adds arm swings and counts faster, Todd enjoys the extra challenge.	Collin lingers at the end of the line as his fellow first-graders practice marching. Even when he chants, "*Hup*, two, three, four," this sensory fumbler can't seem to coordinate his knees in a rhythmic pattern. Adding arm swings and moving faster make it all too frustrating. Collin shuffles along and mutters, "I can't do that."

Emotional Security

Proprioception contributes to our emotional security by orienting us to where our various body parts are and what we are doing with our bodies. The child with poor proprioception is not confident about his own body. Because he lacks the "feel" of it, he is emotionally insecure.

HOW EMOTIONAL SECURITY AFFECTS A CHILD'S BEHAVIOR

A Typical Child	A Child with Proprioceptive Dysfunction
Jenny, five, gets out of bed, dresses, walks to school, does her worksheets, plays outside, and goes on errands with her mother. She feels good about herself and the world she inhabits. Her sense of security results, in part, from dependable messages coming from her body. She can easily orient her body, and this ability gives her confidence as she moves through her day.	For Sara, five, almost everything she does requires effort—getting out of bed, dressing, walking to school, doing her worksheets, playing at the playground, and going on errands with her mother. She doesn't feel good about herself or the world she inhabits. Her sense of insecurity results from the undependable messages coming from her body, which doesn't move the way she wants it to. She has little self-confidence.

CHARACTERISTICS OF PROPRIOCEPTIVE DYSFUNCTION

These checklists will help you gauge whether your child has proprioceptive dysfunction. As you check recognizable characteristics, you will begin to see emerging patterns that explain your child's out-of-sync behavior.

The child who is **overresponsive** to proprioceptive input may:

☐ Prefer not to move.

☐ Become upset when limbs are passively moved.

☐ Become upset when it is necessary to stretch or contract his muscles.

☐ Avoid weight-bearing activities, such as jumping, hopping, running, crawling, rolling, and other physical actions that bring strong proprioceptive input to muscles.

☐ Be a picky eater.

The **underresponsive** child may:

☐ Have low tone.

☐ "Fix" elbow to ribs when writing, or knees tightly together when standing, to compensate for low muscle tone.

☐ Break toys easily.

The **sensory seeking** child may:

☐ Deliberately "bump and crash" into objects in the environment, e.g., jump from high places, dive into a leaf pile, and tackle people.

☐ Stamp or slap his feet on ground when walking.

☐ Kick his heels against the floor or chair.

☐ Bang a stick or other object on a wall or fence while walking.

☐ To modulate his arousal level, engage in self-stimulatory activities, such as head banging, nail biting, finger sucking, or knuckle cracking.

☐ Rub his hands repeatedly on tables.

☐ Like to be tightly swaddled in a blanket or tucked in tightly at bedtime.

☐ Prefer shoelaces, hoods, and belts to be tightly fastened.

☐ Chew constantly on objects, such as shirt collars and cuffs, hood strings, pencils, toys, and gum. The child may enjoy chewy foods.

☐ Appear to be aggressive.

The child with **poor discrimination** and **dyspraxia** may:

☐ Have poor body awareness and motor control.

☐ Have difficulty planning and executing movement. Controlling and monitoring motor tasks such as adjusting a collar or putting on eyeglasses may be especially hard if the child cannot see what he is doing.

☐ Have difficulty positioning his body, as when someone is helping him into a coat, or when he is trying to dress or undress himself.

☐ Have difficulty knowing where his body is in relation to objects and people, frequently falling, tripping, and bumping into obstacles.

☐ Have difficulty going up and down stairs.

☐ Show fear when moving in space.

The child with inefficient **grading of movement** may:

☐ Flex and extend his muscles more or less than necessary for tasks such as inserting his arms into sleeves, or climbing.

☐ Hold pencils and crayons too lightly to make a clear impression, or so tightly that the points break.

☐ Produce messy written work, often with large erasure holes.

☐ Frequently break delicate objects, and seem like a "bull in a china shop."

☐ Break items that require simple manipulation, such as

lamp switches, hair barrettes, and toys that require putting together and pulling apart.

☐ Pick up an object with more force than necessary, such as a glass of milk, causing the object to fly through the air.

☐ Pick up an object with less force than necessary—and thus be unable to lift it. He may complain that objects such as boots or toys are "too heavy."

☐ Have difficulty lifting or holding objects if they don't weigh the same. He may not understand concepts of "heavy" and "light."

The child with sensory-based **postural disorder** may:

☐ Have poor posture.

☐ Lean his head on his hands when he works at a desk.

☐ Slump in a chair, over a table, or while seated on the floor.

☐ Sit on the edge of the chair and keep one foot on the floor for extra stability.

☐ Be unable to keep his balance while standing on one foot.

The child with **emotional insecurity** may:

☐ Avoid participation in ordinary movement experiences, because they make him feel uncomfortable or inadequate.

☐ Become rigid, sticking to the activities that he has mastered and resisting new physical challenges.

☐ Lack self-confidence, saying, "I can't do that," even before trying.

☐ Become timid in unfamiliar situations.

Proprioceptive dysfunction usually coexists with problems with the tactile sense (Chapter Three) and/or vestibular dysfunction (Chapter Four).

Chapter Six

How to Tell if Your Child Has a Problem with the Visual Sense

Two Seventh-Graders at School

Few would guess that Francesca, twelve, has a visual dysfunction. She is the best reader in the seventh grade and loves literature, such as *A Tale of Two Cities*. All she ever does is read, read, read.

Today, after a quick lunch, she scurries from the cafeteria and heads for the library, her haven. She ducks to avoid other students darting through the busy corridor. She enters the library, locates a couple of titles about kites, and goes to an interior corner of the room. Sinking to the floor, she leans against a bookcase, faces the blank wall, and buries her nose in the books.

Francesca loves the tranquil library, where she doesn't squint or get headaches. The reason is that the library has full-spectrum light bulbs in the ceiling, unlike the flickering fluorescent lights in classrooms. Also, in her quiet corner, no sunlight glimmering through venetian blinds can irritate her eyes.

Along comes Charity, also with undetected visual dysfunction, looking for Francesca. Oblivious to most obstacles, Charity bumps into a book cart. The cart tips over; books go flying. She clumsily gathers the books and shoves them onto the cart.

Charity is often confused about where she is in space and has a poor sense of direction. Paying attention to words on the page or moving her eyes smoothly from one line to the next is also hard. Her strength is listening, so she does well in French and Spanish, poetry, and music. Charity is "smart as the Dickens," as Francesca says, but not much of a reader.

Francesca hears Charity coming. "Hi!" she says, glancing up at her friend.

Charity has asked Francesca to scan the shelves for some titles, because that detailed visual job befuddles her. She whispers, "Did you find some good kite books? Any awesome designs?"

"Here's a butterfly pattern for you," Francesca says, "and here's the Baltimore oriole I want to copy." The girls admire the illustrations and whisper about the kites they will be crafting in art class. They are looking forward to an upcoming field trip to Washington, DC, to see the Cherry Blossom Festival parade and to fly kites on the National Mall.

Later, in art class, they attempt to work on their kites and immediately run into problems. One problem is shifting their gaze from the book illustrations to their work and back again. Focusing and refocusing are hard. Another difficulty is transposing the designs they have chosen onto the kite wings. They cannot visualize how to enlarge the butterfly and bird because relating the parts to the whole is a visual skill they have not yet developed.

The art teacher comes to their table and frowns at the girls' cockeyed efforts. She looks for something positive to say. "I see you are both working really hard."

The girls stare at her anxiously. Charity wonders if the teacher is angry. Searching her face, she is not sure.

"Hmm," the teacher says. "Next time, how about if you start over with something less complex? Sometimes, less is more."

"Yes," agrees Charity. "Something simpler." She relaxes a bit. Maybe the teacher is not mad. At least, she doesn't sound mad.

Francesca sighs. "I guess I could just paint big dots, instead of a bird."

The bell rings, and as the girls pack up to leave, the teacher gives them an understanding smile. She cannot understand, however, why such smart pupils struggle over an art project that ought to be well within their capability. Why can't Francesca and Charity make sense of images right before their eyes?

Atypical Patterns of Behavior

Why, indeed, can't Francesca and Charity make sense of what they see?

They both show atypical patterns of behavior. Francesca is overresponsive to visual sensations. Her body's way to compensate is with overaccommodation (a problem with a basic visual skill). Yes, she can read well, but most visual stimulation puts her on overload. She has difficulty negotiating her way through a busy hallway, tolerating flickering light and maintaining direct eye contact.

Charity is underresponsive to visual stimuli. She has difficulty knowing what she is looking at, where it is in space, and where she is in relation to it. One problem is compression of visual attention; she can focus on just one object at a time rather than see the whole picture. Compressed attention causes poor visual figure-ground (a discrimination problem). She cannot make sense of the cart in her path, titles on the bookshelf, and print on the page. She also misreads visual cues in facial expressions.

Additionally, both girls have visual dyspraxia. Their brains are inefficient at integrating visual input with motor output. Thus, their visual-motor responses are delayed and clumsy. They cannot easily use vision to guide their movements and carry out a plan, such as reproducing designs from the book illustrations.

On the next pages you will learn how the visual sense is supposed to function, followed by an explanation of the types of dysfunction that dim these seventh graders' view of the world.

THE SMOOTHLY FUNCTIONING
VISUAL SENSE

Vision is a complex sensory system that enables us to identify sights, anticipate what is "coming at us," and prepare for a response. We use vision, first, to detect contrast, edge, and movement so we can defend ourselves; and second, to guide and direct our movement so we can interact meaningfully in our environment, socialize, and learn.

The stimulus that triggers vision is light, or a change in light. This stimulus is external, and we have no actual physical contact with it, as we do with tactile, vestibular, and proprioceptive stimuli.

A unique feature of vision is providing both temporal (time) and spatial (space) information. We see things sequentially and, at the same time, see a volume of space. For instance, when we read, we move our eyes from one group of words to the next. As we move our eyes to a new position we see and take in another group of words. Vision lets us process an enormous volume of space, in the wink of an eye.

That vision is so important to us now is astounding, because, in terms of evolution, vision is a newcomer to the nervous system. Smell was the dominant sense of our ancient ancestors and still is crucial for many animals. Today, vision is humankind's dominant sense for learning where we are and what is happening around us, or what may happen at any moment.

Vision should not be confused with eyesight, which is only one part of vision. Eyesight, the basic ability to see the big "E" on the wall chart, is a given. Eyesight is a prerequisite for vision. Either we see, or we don't. We can neither learn nor be taught to see.

INTERESTING FACTS ABOUT VISION

• 80 percent of the information we take in comes through the eyes.

• 80 percent of visual processing is responsible for what we see, and 20 percent is responsible for where and how we see.

• 66-$\frac{2}{3}$ percent of the brain activity of the brain is devoted to vision when the eyes are open. Three billion impulses come into the CNS every second; two billion of these are visual.

• 93 percent of human communication is nonverbal; 55 percent of communication comes from seeing the speaker's facial expressions and body gestures.

• 75–90 percent of classroom learning depends on vision.

• 90 percent of visual problems are never diagnosed.

• 25 percent of all school-age students have undiagnosed vision problems.

• 70 percent of juvenile delinquents have undiagnosed vision problems.

Vision, unlike sight, is not a skill we are born with but rather one we develop gradually as we integrate our senses. Growing up, we learn to make sense of what we see.

How? Through movement! Movement, the basis of all learning, teaches the eyes to make sense of sights, whereas sitting still to read or to gaze at the computer screen does not.

The vestibular and proprioceptive systems profoundly influence our vision. When we stretch and contract postural muscles to lie down, sit up, or stand on two feet, sensations bombard our brain and facilitate eye movements. When we move around, switch directions, and change the position of our body, head, and eyes, we strengthen visual skills. When we engage in purposeful activity, our eyes become better coordinated. Thus, movement, balance, muscle control, and postural responses are "must haves" for proper vision development.

The tactile sense, too, has a huge effect on vision. The infant's hand grazes his toes, and he turns to see what he has touched. The preschooler handles an orange and pays visual attention to its tactile properties. Tomorrow he can see another orange and know that it is round, rough, solid, and just right for holding, squeezing, rolling and tossing. The older student can visualize images, such as a pyramid, a policeman, or a pepperoni pizza without touching or seeing the real thing. To see well, countless, concrete, tactile experiences really count!

The auditory sense affects vision, as well. When we hear a sound, the auditory information reinforces our visual processing about its whereabouts. A door slams, a friend calls our name, or a bird warbles; we turn to locate and see the source of the sound. Also, hearing reinforces our visual processing about what is being said. For example, hearing or saying the word "apple" triggers a visual image of an apple.

Indeed, we need all our senses to develop vision, just as we need vision to develop the other senses—including smell and taste. The ability to know many sensory details about what we see, such as a muffin's aroma and flavor, even before we eat it, is the happy result of sensory integration.

Two Components: Defensive ("Okay!" or "Uh, Oh!") and Discriminative ("Aha!")

Like the other senses, vision has two components. Our first response is always defensive (see Chapter Two). Vision acts primarily to protect us from danger. When light hits the eye, our immediate response is reflexive, i.e., involuntary and without conscious control. Automatically, we make adaptive responses so we can see clearly, for clear and single vision is an essential survival skill.

Basic visual skills—the unconscious mechanisms of sight—include:

- Acuity, the ability to see details of objects.

- Adjusting from dark to bright light, e.g., when we step from a dim hall into the sun.

- Accommodation in each eye so we can focus on objects at varying distances, both at far point and at near point, such as looking back and forth from the desk to a scene outside the window or copying problems from the chalkboard into an assignment notebook.

- Detection of movement, such as the spider creeping up the wall, the car coming down the road, or classmates moving in the schoolroom.

- Binocularity (two-eyed vision), the ability to sweep the eyes together in a coordinated way and use them as a team to form a single mental picture from the images that the eyes separately record, such as looking skyward with two eyes to see just one moon.

- Ocular-motor (eye motor) skills, including steady attention on an object (fixation), efficient movement from point to point or word to word (saccades), and tracking of a moving object (smooth pursuits), such as a ball in the air.

With healthy, working eyes as the foundation, we can get on with the discriminative component of vision, involving conscious, higher level cognitive functions. (Various terms are used for these functions, including "visual-spatial perception," "visual cognition," "spatial cognition," "form and space perception," and "visual discrimination," the term used here.)

Visual discrimination helps us refine details about what we see, where that object is in space, and where we are in relation to it. This "what, where, and how" of vision guides our responses to what we see.

HOW BASIC VISUAL SKILLS
AFFECT A CHILD'S BEHAVIOR

A Typical Child	A Child with Poor Visual Skills
Mason, thirteen, lives for baseball. He is a "physical genius," his coach says, in part because of his excellent visual skills. Up at bat, he easily keeps his eyes on the ball and shifts his focus quickly from a far point (outfielder Kerry) to a near point (home plate). When he pitches, good eye-teaming helps him see exactly where to place the ball. He is a natural.	Until Kerry, an eighth-grader, got glasses and vision therapy, he was not a notable ball player. Now, up at bat, fixing his gaze on the pitcher and tracking fast balls is easier. When Kerry is in the outfield, he no longer strains to coordinate his eye movements. When he is very tired, he may still see double, but most of the time he is one of the team's most valuable players.

Discriminative skills include:

• Peripheral vision—awareness of images that surround us through the sides of our eyes, primarily for detecting motion.

• Depth perception—seeing objects and spaces around oneself in three dimensions and judging relative distances between objects, or between oneself and objects, in order to descend the stairs and avoid stepping on cracks in the pavement.

• Stable visual field—discerning which objects move and which objects remain stationary.

• Spatial relationships—including directionality (judging how close objects are to other objects and to oneself) and laterality (with one's own two-sidedness as a reference, the awareness of right/left, front/back and up/down).

• Visual discrimination—discerning likenesses and differences in size, shape, pattern, form, position, and color.

• Form constancy—recognition of a form, symbol, or shape even when its size, position, or texture changes, in order to match, separate, or categorize objects, or to know whether a letter is "u" or "n," or "p" or "q."

• Visual figure-ground—differentiating objects in the foreground and background, to distinguish one word on a page, or a face in a crowd.

• Visual attention—using the eyes, brain, and body together long enough to stay with an activity, such as reading, following directions, or looking at an object or person.

• Visual memory—recognizing, associating, storing, and retrieving visual details that one has seen previously.

• Sequential memory—perceiving words and pictures in order and remembering the sequence, important for reading and spelling.

• Visualization—forming and manipulating images of objects, people, or scenarios in one's mind's eye, a prerequisite for language development.

• Visual-sensory integration, combining vision with touch, movement, balance, posture, hearing, and other sensory messages.

With both components of vision in sync, we not only see, but also respond adaptively to what we see in social and physical surroundings. Visual-motor skills are movements based on the discrimination of visual information. These skills gradually evolve, and we learn to connect seeing with doing, or praxis. After much practice, we can coordinate the "what, where, and how" of vision with gross-motor and fine-motor movement. Is our sock covered with lint? We can pick it off. Is the pothole deep and wide? We can move around it. Visual-motor skills include:

• Eye-hand coordination—the ability of the eyes to guide fine-motor tasks, such as manipulating toys, fitting round pegs into round holes, using tools, eating, dressing, writing, and following printed patterns to lace beads or build block structures.

• Eye-foot coordination—the ability of the eyes to guide gross-motor activities such as playing hopscotch, stepping into the bathtub, and kicking a ball.

• Eye-ear coordination—the ability of the eyes to see a letter, integrate the message with stored auditory information, and tell a person how to say it or use it in a word.

The child who has developed visual discrimination and visual-motor skills has had much practice in looking around, moving around, and actively participating in a variety of sensory experiences. This child can judge accurately where objects are in space and can build a block tower or visualize an elegant bridge design in 3-D. He can recognize a hammer, an "R," and a trapezoid, whether it is right-side up or upside down. In his schoolwork, he can line up columns of numbers and write neatly between the margins. He can move fluidly across a room or playing field. He can travel in the same direction as everyone else in a parade. He can ride a bike from garage to grocery store and draw, read, and follow a treasure map.

An Example of Visual Skills at Work

Envision this scenario to understand how important all the components of vision are for survival: You are walking on the sidewalk beside the green park and notice a diagonal path cutting through to the opposite side. You veer off the sidewalk and take the path (directionality). You sweep your eyes (binocularity) from left to right (scanning) and sense that the park environment is peaceful. From the corner of your eye (peripheral vision), you espy a slight motion (detection of movement) coming from a big lump wrapped in a red blanket and lying on a bench (visual discrimination). You freeze so the lump won't notice you. From afar, you evaluate the scene. Could that lump be a person lying down (form constancy)? It looks like other lumps you have seen (visual memory). You focus so your vision won't be blurred (accommodation). You gaze at the lump, the bench, the tree, and the path (fixation) and concentrate on the whole scene (visual attention). Is this situation good for you, bad for you, or neutral? Where is the lump in relation to where you are and where are you relative to safety on the busy street (spatial relationships)? Can you find your way out of the park (wayfinding)? The lump stirs suddenly, and you jump (visual defensiveness). Without hesitating to analyze whether to fight it, flee from it, feed on it, feed it, or mate with it, you make a self-protective adaptive response. You simply point your feet in the opposite direction and run (eye-foot coordination).

THE OUT-OF-SYNC VISUAL SENSE

Dr. Ayres and her gifted followers have found that many children with learning disabilities have visual dysfunction. Usually, their brains are inefficient in coordinating visual discrimination and visual-motor skills with vestibular, proprioceptive, and postural mechanisms. In other words, their eyes and bodies are out of sync.

Erratic vision development is common in children with autism—although often it is overlooked. The child with autism often has poor eye contact and has difficulty attending to and giving meaning to objects and people in his environment. When he is visually stressed, he may squint and "self-stim" (flap his hands in front of his eyes). "Self-stimming" is a compensatory attempt to open up visual space, relax his compressed visual attention, and function better.

Of course, many children without autism have obvious or not-so-obvious visual dysfunction, too. When dysfunction involves movement (tripping on air), posture (slumping at the desk), and body awareness (difficulty learning left and right), then chances are that the problem is sensory based, and SPD is the root.

However, when dysfunction involves visual discrimination without movement (such as matching colors or reading a map), SPD is not necessarily the root. The cause could be an acuity problem, such as nearsightedness, or a cognitive disorder, such as Down Syndrome. Determining the underlying cause of visual problems matters greatly so that the appropriate treatment will match the specific problem.

The child with SPD and poor vision may have one or more problems with modulating, discriminating, and using visual sensations to respond adaptively to the world.

Sensory Modulation Disorders

VISUAL OVERRESPONSIVITY—"OH, NO!"

The child with overresponsivity, or visual defensiveness, reacts dramatically to benign environmental stimuli such as contrasts, reflections, shiny surfaces, and bright lights. She may turn her eyes away from sudden, vivid, or flickering lights, perhaps shielding her eyes with her hands, sunglasses, or a cap visor. The child may also

HOW OVERRESPONSIVITY
AFFECTS A CHILD'S BEHAVIOR

A Typical Child	A Child with Visual Overresponsivity
Leah, eleven, is looking after her little brother at the playground. He toddles toward the swings. In the nick of time, Leah notices that he is in the direct path of a child swinging down in a wide arc. Without hesitation, she grabs her brother's arm and tugs him out of the way.	Dorothy, eleven, baby-sits for a neighbor. At the park, the toddler tugs Dorothy toward the swings. The rapid movement of the children on the swings alarms her. She closes her eyes to avoid the commotion. One of the swingers inadvertently knocks her and her little charge to the ground.

be disturbed by moving objects, such as dangling mobiles or people bustling in a busy environment. She may duck when objects come toward her, such as a ball or another fast-moving child.

VISUAL UNDERRESPONSIVITY—"HO, HUM"

The underresponsive child may not pay attention to novel visual stimuli, such as holiday decorations or rearranged classroom furniture. She may not respond quickly and efficiently when objects come toward her—for example, when a beanbag is tossed her way.

HOW UNDERRESPONSIVITY
AFFECTS A CHILD'S BEHAVIOR

A Typical Child	A Child with Visual Underresponsivity
Connor, a fourth-grader, looks up at the homework assignment chalked on the blackboard. He copies the assignment in his notebook, glances up again to compare it to what he wrote to be sure he got it right, gathers his gear into his backpack, and heads for the door.	While other children copy the assignment from the board, Rex, nine, stares out the window. The teacher beckons him and says, "It may be easier to hear the assignment than to read it. I'll tell you what to write down." Rex is grateful but can't hold her gaze. He stares right through her.

She may be unaware of bright light or sun. She may not blink or turn away from the dazzling light. She may stare at objects without seeming to see them, or at people's faces as if they are not even there.

SENSORY SEEKING—"MORE!"

The child who seeks more visual stimulation than most children may clamor for excessive time in front of the television or computer screen, and may be attracted to bright, flickering lights, such as strobe lights or stripes of sunlight pouring through window blinds.

HOW SENSORY SEEKING
AFFECTS A CHILD'S BEHAVIOR

A Typical Child	*A Sensory Craver*
The defective fluorescent light slightly annoys Lucy, four, but she ignores it during Show and Tell. Then, it is time to play outdoors. After school, she goes to Lynne's. She joins Lynne briefly to watch a video until she gets bored and looks for some dress-ups to try on.	Lynne, four, gazes up at the flickering fluorescent light. The long "on" and brief "off" distract her from Show and Tell. After school, Lucy comes to her house to play. Lynne sits close to the TV and stares at a mesmerizing video, while Lucy slips away and tries on dress-ups.

Poor Visual Discrimination

The typical child can distinguish specific qualities about what she sees and can tell the difference between the people and things she looks at.

The child with poor visual discrimination does not perceive what he sees. Instead of linking visual information with auditory, touch, and movement sensations, his brain may misconnect the messages. For instance, if connecting sights with sounds is a problem, he may not know where to look when he hears the teacher's voice. If connecting sights with touch sensations is a problem, he may not know—just by looking—that a nail is sharp and a hammer is heavy. If connecting sights with movement sensations is a problem, he may not swerve to avoid bumping into furniture. If all the sensory pieces don't come together in his brain into a unified whole, it is most challenging to adapt responsively to the sights his eyes record.

The child may be unable to match or separate colors, shapes, numbers, letters, and words. He may not distinguish words in print, even his own name. As he grows, he may stumble over similar symbols, letters, and numbers, such as ▲ and ▼, "b" and "d," and *1,000* and *1,000,000*. He may have difficulty focusing and concentrating

165

HOW VISUAL DISCRIMINATION
AFFECTS A CHILD'S BEHAVIOR

A Typical Child	A Child with Poor Visual Discrimination
Samantha, five, is studying a magazine page called, "What's Wrong with this Picture?" She spots an upside-down "4" on a kitchen clock, a banana where a telephone receiver should be, and a tiny spider in a line of ants marching toward a sugar bowl. Giggling, she tries to share the page with Opal, but Opal's inattention disappoints her.	Opal, a kindergartner with visual dysfunction, looks briefly at "What's Wrong with this Picture?" when Samantha shows it to her. But Opal cannot easily pick out the visual details, so the page does not hold her attention. She shrugs and hands it back to Samantha. She does not recognize Samantha's disappointment.

on details in pictures, puzzles, Lego instructions, history books, geometric proofs, recipes, sewing patterns, and so forth.

The child may be unsuccessful at differentiating between objects in the foreground and in the background. He may not enjoy examining richly illustrated books such as *Where's Waldo?* He may misjudge which jigsaw pieces fit into a puzzle and be unable to spot a friend in a crowd.

He may misread important visual cues in social interactions, such as facial expressions and gestures, which make up more than half of our human communication. The inability to discriminate whether another person is scowling or smiling is a significant disadvantage!

Visual-Motor Skills

The typical child uses visual information to guide her planned and purposeful movement. With synchronized visual-motor skills, she can move her body efficiently, get from Point A to Point B, look at and copy a simple drawing or block structure, and see, reach for, and grasp an object.

The child with poor visual-motor skills has difficulty using her vision to guide her movements. Visual dyspraxia may cause problems in visualizing, planning, and carrying out a sequence of complex movements, such as rolling over in bed to see the alarm clock. She may overreach for objects. She may stumble up stairs. She may find it hard to walk on a balance beam, ride a bicycle, tie shoes, cut out paper dolls, spread butter on toast, or thread a needle. She may be bewildered, emotionally insecure, and "lost in space."

Poor eye-hand coordination may mean the child struggles to use his eyes and hands together. He may have difficulty manipulating toys and school materials, catching balls, using crayons and pencils, and fastening his clothes.

Poor eye-foot coordination will impede a child's smooth walking, running, and success on the playing field. Poor eye-ear coordination will interfere with his ability to see and then say a letter or word, and thus, with his speaking, reading and writing skills.

HOW EYE-HAND COORDINATION
AFFECTS A CHILD'S BEHAVIOR

A Typical Child	*A Child with Poor Eye-Hand Coordination*
At snack time, David, three, pours juice into a cup, stopping just before the juice reaches the brim. After snack, he works on a puzzle. One piece doesn't seem to fit. He studies it and realizes that it is upside down. He corrects his error and completes the puzzle. Then he does another, more complicated one.	At snack time, Freddy pours juice until the cup overflows. The teacher cleans him up and offers him a simple jigsaw puzzle. Freddy attempts to put in the four pieces but can't get them to fit. Frustrated, he shoves the puzzle off the table. He asks just to sit in the cozy corner and hold the guinea pig.

The child with visual dyspraxia may be unable to plan ahead and solve problems in his mind's eye. He may look at materials, know something can be done with them, and be unable to recruit the visual functions and skills needed to make something desirable actually happen.

HOW VISUAL PRAXIS AFFECTS A CHILD'S BEHAVIOR

A Typical Child	A Child with Visual Dyspraxia
Herbie and Curt, second-graders, are playing with toy soldiers. Herbie's idea is to map out a battlefield in the sandbox, add pebbles and twigs, and arrange their armies in strategic positions. As the work progresses, he visualizes how to place his men strategically—some behind a rock, others between leafy branches, and others behind sand hills. This is exciting and engrossing work.	Curt agrees that a battlefield in the sandbox is a good idea, but he has no design or strategy in mind. He has difficulty sequencing and using visual information well. He lets Herbie propose and carry out his plan. Curt's side of the battleground is mostly open territory. He lines up his soldiers in parallel rows and waits for the battle to begin.

Poor bilateral integration and poor postural responses frequently interfere with visual-motor skills. The child may have difficulty coordinating both sides of the body and stabilizing his head, trunk, and limbs to function effectively and to support visual-motor skills.

HOW POSTURAL RESPONSES AFFECT A CHILD'S BEHAVIOR

A Typical Child	A Child with Postural Disorder
At his table, Benjamin, a first-grader, sits upright and reads the workbook instructions. He understands them, picks up his crayon, and connects the dots.	Clark, six, slumps at the table. He twists on the chair, trying to get comfortable so he can read the workbook. He cocks his head this way and that. The words dance on the page.

Fortunately, help is available. A developmental optometrist can provide vision therapy to strengthen eye-motor control, visual discrimination, and eye-hand coordination (see Chapter Eight).

Also, when occupational therapists provide therapy using a sensory integration framework to alleviate vestibular, proprioceptive, and postural problems, vision often improves. If therapy is not an option, a sensory diet rich in visual experiences is essential to ensure adequate vision development. To move is to see!

CHARACTERISTICS OF
VISUAL DYSFUNCTION

These checklists will help you gauge whether your child has visual dysfunction. As you check recognizable characteristics, you will begin to see emerging patterns that help to explain your child's out of sync behavior.

The child with a problem with **basic visual skills** may:

- ☐ Have headaches, eye strain, or red, burning, itchy, or teary eyes.
- ☐ Rub eyes or blink, frown, and squint excessively.
- ☐ Complain about blurred images when looking at pictures, print, or faces.
- ☐ Complain of seeing double.
- ☐ Complain that words seem to move on the page.
- ☐ Turn or tilt her head as she reads across a page.
- ☐ Hold a book too closely, or lower her face too closely to the desk.
- ☐ Have difficulty seeing the storybook or chalkboard, and request to move nearer.

☐ Have difficulty shifting her gaze from one object to another, such as when looking from the blackboard to her own paper, and make errors in copying.

☐ Have difficulty focusing on stationary objects.

☐ Frequently lose her place on the page, reread words or lines, and omit numbers, letters, words, or lines when reading or writing, and need to use her finger to keep her place.

☐ Have difficulty tracking or following a moving object, such as a ping-pong ball, or following along a line of printed words.

☐ Fatigue easily during schoolwork and sports-related activities.

The child with difficulty **modulating visual sensations** may:

☐ Shield her eyes to screen out sights, close or cover one eye, or squint.

☐ Avoid bright lights and sunlight, perhaps preferring to wear sunglasses, even indoors.

☐ Be uncomfortable or overwhelmed by moving objects or people.

☐ Duck or try to avoid objects coming toward her, such as a ball or another child.

☐ Withdraw from classroom participation and avoid group-movement activities.

☐ Avoid direct eye contact.

☐ Experience headaches, nausea, or dizziness when using eyes.

☐ Be unaware of light/dark contrast, edges, and reflections.

☐ Be unaware of movement, often bumping into moving objects such as swings.

☐ Respond late to visual information, such as obstacles in her path.

☐ Seek bright lights, strobe lights, and direct sunlight.

☐ Seek visual stimulation, such as finger flicking, spinning, and peering at patterns and edges, such as ceiling and fence lines.

☐ Move excessively (squirm, fidget) during visual tasks, such as workbook activities.

The child with poor **visual discrimination** may:

☐ Have difficulty seeing objects in three dimensions (depth perception).

☐ Seem overwhelmed by moving objects or people because of a problem discriminating between what moves and what is motionless (stable visual field).

☐ Have difficulty judging relative distances between objects, such as letters, words, numbers, or drawings on a page; between oneself and objects in the environment, often bumping into things (spatial relationships).

☐ Not understand concepts such as up/down, forward/ back, before/after, and first/second. The child may have a problem stringing beads in order, following a pattern to build with blocks, or wayfinding (going from one place to another without getting lost, or finding one's way in a new place).

☐ Have difficulty in team sports that require awareness of position on the field or court and knowledge of teammates' positions and movements.

☐ Confuse likenesses and differences in pictures, words, symbols, and objects and have difficulty distinguishing properties of objects.

☐ Repeatedly confuse similar beginnings and endings of words ("tree/three," "fight/flight/fright," "window/ winter").

☐ Have difficulty with schoolwork involving the size of letters, the spacing of letters and words on the line, and the lining up of numbers (form constancy). The child may reverse letters ("b/d") or words ("saw/was") while reading and writing.

☐ Have difficulty differentiating objects in the foreground and background, necessary to distinguish one word on a page, or a face in a crowd (visual figure-ground).

☐ Be unable to form mental images of objects, people, or scenarios, to envision what she reads or hears, or relate pictures and words to the "real thing" (visualization).

☐ Have difficulty describing thoughts and actions, both verbally and in writing.

☐ Be a poor speller.

☐ Have difficulty remembering what he did or saw during the day.

☐ Be unable to interpret how objects would feel, just by looking at them; the child must touch the kitten to know it is soft and furry.

☐ Fail to comprehend what she is reading, or quickly lose interest.

☐ Have a short attention span for reading or copying information from the board, and have a poor visual memory of what she read.

The child with poor **visual-motor skills** may:

☐ Have poor eye-hand coordination—the efficient teamwork of the eyes and hands, necessary for playing with toys, using tools, dressing, writing, and academic tasks.

☐ Be unable to use her eyes to guide hand movements necessary for accurate orientation of drawings and words on a page. She may be unable to stay within the lines when she colors, and her writing may be crooked and poorly spaced.

☐ Have difficulty with fine-motor tasks involving spatial relationships, such as doing jigsaw puzzles, rearranging dollhouse furniture, and cutting along lines.

☐ Have poor eye-foot coordination and difficulty walking upstairs or kicking balls.

☐ Have poor gross-motor skills and difficulty moving on playground equipment, such as reaching for and climbing on monkey bars.

☐ Avoid sports and group activities in which movement is required.

☐ Have difficulty with rhythmic activities.

☐ Have poor coordination and balance.

☐ Have difficulty sounding out a word silently and then saying it, or she may mispronounce similar words as she continues reading (eye-ear coordination).

☐ Orient drawings poorly on the page, or write uphill or downhill.

☐ Have exceedingly poor posture while at the table or desk, or twist in an unusual way to see the teacher or book.

☐ Withdraw from classroom participation.

☐ Have low self-esteem.

Chapter Seven

How to Tell if Your Child Has a Problem with the Auditory Sense

A Third-Grader in Music Class

This is the first Monday after vacation, and May has a stomach ache. She doesn't want to go to school, because on Mondays the third-graders go to the all-purpose room for music. May hates the teacher, crabby old Miss Cross, who insists that the children sit still during the whole lesson. She is not attuned to children like May who learn best by moving.

The children are practicing for the spring concert. When they come into the room, first they sit and sing folk songs. May mouths the words without voicing them, because Miss Cross told her, "If you won't sing in tune, don't sing out loud." Miss Cross doesn't understand that May would sing in tune if she could, but she can't.

After singing, the children play instruments. Half the students play the tunes on their recorders, while the others accompany them on drums, rhythm sticks, and other unpitched percussion instruments. Then the groups switch and repeat the repertoire.

May hates the recorder because she never knows if the note she plays sounds as it should. She does not have good pitch, the highness or lowness of sounds in relation to one another. She may try to play B, for instance, but her recorder sometimes squawks out a tone that is too sharp and sounds higher, like C. The other kids sidle away, and Miss Cross glares.

Playing the unpitched instruments is somewhat easier, but May also has problems with rhythm, timing, and dynamics. She comes in late, can't catch or keep the beat, and plays *fortissimo* when she should play *pianissimo*. May just doesn't "get it" when it comes to making music.

Today, the children enter the room and are surprised to see a new teacher. Mr. Harmon smiles as they sit down. He says, "I'm your teacher now. Miss Cross decided not to come back after vacation. She gave me some tips about managing this class, but I'm going to toss those tips out the window and do something different. Let's get our whole bodies into this music-making business. Everybody, up! Let's move!"

Instead of making the children sit, he has them stand in one spot and sing scales, bending to touch the floor and stretching toward the ceiling to match the ascending and descending notes. Then they move around the room singing songs. He instructs them to walk and sing slowly, run and sing fast, stomp and sing loudly, tiptoe and sing softly.

May watches the other children for a moment until she catches on. Once she gets moving, she loves the crouching, stretching, and locomotion. She is not merely hearing the music— she is incorporating it into her body. It's all beginning to make sense.

Finally, with their bodies and voices primed, the children pick up the instruments. With a new sense of pitch and rhythm in her body, May understands how she can transpose some of that feeling into the music. Playing the recorder isn't so hard today.

Next Monday, May will be eager to go to school. Stomach aches on music day? Unheard of!

Atypical Pattern of Behavior

When processing sounds, May shows an atypical pattern of behavior. Her auditory processing problems are a type of Sensory Discrimination Disorder.

She sings and plays the recorder out of tune, because she cannot discriminate differences in pitch in the musical tones. She is off the beat when playing the percussion instruments, because of her inadequate sense of timing and rhythm. She must look at the other children when following the teacher's directions, because hearing the instructions is not enough—she needs visual information to help her understand what she hears.

Many children with Sensory Discrimination Disorder also have modulation problems, but May does not. (She does not have auditory defensiveness; she is not oblivious to sounds; and she does not crave loud and constant noise.) She is somewhat clumsy, but once she understands Mr. Harmon's expectations, her body movements and motor planning improve.

THE SMOOTHLY FUNCTIONING
AUDITORY SENSE

The vestibular and auditory systems work together as they process sensations of movement and sound. These sensations are closely intertwined, because they both begin to be processed by hair cells in the receptors of the ear.

Hearing, or audition, is the ability to receive sounds. We are born with this basic skill. We can't learn how to do it; either we hear, or we don't.

Auditory skills begin developing in the womb. The auditory nervous system is the first to become functional. In tandem with the vestibular system, it connects with muscles throughout the body and helps to regulate movement, equilibrium, and coordination.

The ear's influence on physical development is profound.

Indeed, the ear is vital not only for hearing, balance, and flexibility, but also for bilateral coordination, respiration (breathing), speaking, self-esteem, social relationships, vision, and, of course, academic learning.

Two Components: Defensive ("Okay!" or "Uh, Oh!") and Discriminative ("Aha!")

The auditory sense, like the other senses, begins with a defensive component. As babies, we startle when we hear loud or unexpected noise. Gradually, our brains develop the ability to modulate sensations and tell us whether the sound is one we can enjoy and use or must avoid for self-protection. When we realize that a sound was just a door shutting, and not a danger, we return to a state of being calm and alert.

The abilities to hear and to modulate sensations of sound underlie our ability to really listen to sounds around us and understand their meaning. We are not born with the skill of listening; we acquire it, as we integrate vestibular and auditory sensations. Gradually, as we interact purposefully with our environment, we learn to interpret what we hear and to develop sophisticated auditory discrimination skills.

The discriminative component of the auditory sense evolves as the child moves, touches, and engages in many multisensory experiences. Discriminative functions, which help us refine details about the "what" and "where" of sounds, include:

- Localization—the ability to identify the source of a sound, such as a parent's voice, or a friend's "Yoo-hoo!"—and to judge the distance between the sound and oneself.

- Tracking—the ability to follow a sound, such as a helicopter as it putters across the sky or someone's footsteps as he patters around the house.

- Auditory memory—the ability to remember what was heard, e.g., conversations, directions, homework assignments, or song lyrics, and to refer to it at once (immediate memory) or later (deferred memory).

• Auditory sequencing—the ability to put in order what was heard and repeat it in logical order, such as the alphabet, Spanish verb conjugations, or multisyllabic words like "obstacle" or "nuclear."

• Auditory discrimination—the ability to compare and contrast environmental sounds, such as a food blender and a vacuum cleaner, and to hear likenesses and differences in word sounds, such as road/load, flute/fruit, cup/cut.

• Auditory figure-ground—the ability to distinguish between foreground and background sounds, in order to hear the main message without being distracted.

• Association—the ability to relate a novel sound to a familiar sound, such as connecting the bark of the neighbor's new puppy to the category of "dog," and the ability to relate a visual symbol, such as an alphabet letter or a musical note, with its particular sound.

• Auditory cohesion—the higher level listening ability to unite various ideas into a coherent whole, to draw inferences from what is said, to understand riddles, jokes, puns, and verbal math problems, and to take notes in class.

• Auditory attention—the ability to maintain focus sufficiently to listen to a teacher's lesson, a conversation, or a story, essential for bringing the other auditory processing skills together.

AN EXAMPLE OF AUDITORY SKILLS AT WORK

You attend Field Day at your child's school. Two hundred adults and children are milling about, talking, and laughing. All around, the decibel level is high, but you get used to it.

Unexpectedly, a P.E. teacher right behind you yells instructions through a bullhorn. You duck and cover your ears. What was he shouting? You aren't sure because you had to shut out the noise. He moves down the sidelines. Aha, now you can listen to his message about lining up by classes (auditory attention). You hear a different sound now—it is a drummer (auditory discrimination) leading the band from the school building toward the crowd (tracking). You find yourself marching to the steady beat (ear body coordination) as you move along the edge of the field. You look for your child but don't see her. Through the din, you hear her calling, "Hi, Mom!" (figure-ground). You turn to the source of the sound (localization), and wave to your child across the field. Then, the band strikes up "The Star Spangled Banner." The crowd hushes. Everyone sings (auditory memory). Another parent says, "Isn't this great?" You nod (receptive language) and reply, "Field Day is always fun!" (expressive language). The games begin.

When defensive and discriminative components are in sync, we can respond adaptively to sounds. We know what the sounds are and where they come from, or can make educated guesses based on previous sounds we have heard. With information about the "what" and "where" of sounds, we develop auditory-motor coordination—what I call "ear-body coordination"—and learn how and when to move in accordance with the sounds. Our infant's hungry cry makes us prepare to nurse. A harsh tirade makes us cringe, rush-hour honking makes us tense, and clear, orderly music, such as Mozart's, makes us alert and organized.

When we process sounds typically, we can put out the uniquely human products of speech and language. Speech and language are entwined but not the same. Speech is the physical production of sound. Speech depends on smoothly functioning muscles in the throat, tongue, lips, and jaw. The vestibular, proprioceptive, and tactile systems govern motor control and motor planning for using those fine muscles to produce intelligible speech.

Language is the meaningful use of words, which are symbols representing objects and ideas. Thus, language is a code for deciphering what words imply and how we use them to relate to others.

Language that we take in and understand, through listening and reading, is called "receptive." Receptive language focuses on external sounds, i.e., voices of other people and the noises all around us.

Language that we put out to communicate, through speaking, singing, or writing, is "expressive." Expressive language focuses on sounds we hear internally and that we reproduce, as accurately as possible, through our own voice.

We listen, move, speak, and read with our ear. Body awareness, balance, motor coordination, muscle control, postural responses, sequencing, language skills, planning ahead, and problem solving grow stronger as we process the sounds that surround us.

THE OUT-OF-SYNC AUDITORY SENSE

An auditory processing problem often occurs along with SPD. However, this problem can also stand alone, as the result, perhaps, of ear infections or hearing loss.

With or without SPD, a child may hear adequately but process sounds slowly or inaccurately. She may have a problem modulating or discriminating sensations of sound. Or she may be dyspraxic and come to a standstill when she hears sounds, not knowing how or when to start or stop an activity. Her rhythm and timing is off, affecting how she moves, reads, and communicates.

Her language may suffer. Recalling what she wants to say, putting her thoughts in order, or getting the words out may be hard. She may have a problem pronouncing words clearly enough to be understood. She may lack awareness of how her mouth, lips, and tongue feel and work together. She may say "tool" instead of "school," or "dese" instead of "these," because of difficulty positioning the muscles necessary for articulation.

Sensory Modulation Disorders

AUDITORY OVERRESPONSIVITY—"OH, NO!"
For most of us, most of the time, when loud noises come at us, a muscle in the middle ear contracts to stifle the vibrations. This mechanism protects us from being overwhelmed or deafened. However, when we feel threatened ("Uh, oh!") and go into fight/flight/freeze mode, this little muscle does not clamp down. Instantly, keen attention to all sounds is imperative.

People whose auditory defensiveness keeps them constantly alert must listen to every sound. Easily distracted, some respond to ordinary noise with an infantile, whole-body startle. This state of ceaseless, on-edge alertness uses up energy, interferes with learning, and hampers language development and social interactions.

People on the autistic spectrum (and others, too, of course) often have auditory overresponsivity, or auditory defensiveness. Sounds that please others, such as chirping birds or rustling leaves, can make them feel as if their eardrums are being scraped.

HOW OVERRESPONSIVITY
AFFECTS A CHILD'S BEHAVIOR

A Typical Child	A Child with Auditory Overresponsivity
Before lunch, Brynna, a fifth-grader, rushes to the school bathroom. The flushing toilets and whirring hand dryers are loud, but these everyday sounds don't bother her. When she hears loud, sudden noises such as screeching tires or fire alarms, she pays attention and winces. Otherwise, she briefly perks up her ears to unexpected sounds, such as books falling off a desk, and then ignores them.	When Nelia, ten, gets home from school, she rushes to the bathroom. She never goes at school because the noise of the toilet hurts her ears. The flushing water is as deafening as Niagara Falls. Nelia also jumps out of her skin and claps her hands over her ears when a pencil hits the floor or a door clicks shut. Her oversensitivity to sounds makes everyone refer to her as "Nervous Nellie."

With or without autism, the sensory avoider reacts strongly, swiftly, and negatively to loud, unexpected noises. He will alert to most sounds—even sounds that are too faint or high-pitched for most people to hear. When he hears sirens blaring, block towers tumbling, or people chewing, he may complain or cover his ears. Indeed, this child may worry incessantly about the possibility of loud noises, and that worry may affect his behavior.

If the metallic twang of guitar strings hurts, he may hang back from sing-alongs. If the sound of a balloon popping distresses him, he may refuse to go to birthday parties. If the rock concert promises a big sound, he may prefer an evening home alone. If he can't get away from the hubbub, he may raise his own voice, hollering, "La-La-La-La!" to counteract noise, rather like fighting fire with fire.

AUDITORY UNDERRESPONSIVITY—"HO, HUM"

The "sensory disregarder" seems unaware of sounds that others hear and listen to. But is the child who seems unaware *truly* unaware? In many cases, we don't know. Children with autism, for example, who cannot express themselves, clearly may sense more than we can detect merely by looking at them.

HOW UNDERRESPONSIVITY
AFFECTS A CHILD'S BEHAVIOR

A Typical Child	*A Child with Auditory Underresponsivity*
At the playground, kindergartners Asher and Frankie are playing with trucks at the base of the monkey bars. Another little boy, Jed, is climbing overhead and prepares to let go. He says, "Look out, look out!" Asher leaps nimbly out of the way, just in the nick of time.	Frankie is crouching under the monkey bars, engrossed with his truck. He hears Jed cry, "Look out!"—but does not respond and continues his play. Jed lets go and lands nearby. Startled, Frankie whimpers, "Don't do that." Jed says, "I told you I was gonna jump, you baby."

The child with underresponsivity to sound does not visibly respond to quiet sounds, soft voices and whispers that may be "under his radar." Likewise, he does not seem to respond to ordinary sounds, voices, questions, and comments. And when he does respond, he may speak very softly, almost in a whisper.

SENSORY SEEKING: THE SENSORY CRAVER— "MORE!"

The "sensory seeker" loves crowds and places with noisy action like rodeos, car races, and parades. He welcomes loud noises and usually wants to turn the volume up. He may make his own noisy sounds, using his "outside voice" in the classroom and kitchen, and clapping and singing boisterously.

A Typical Child	A Child with Sensory Seeking
Thea, seven, is playing at Kaneesha's. Thea covers her ears when her friend turns the TV way up. "Ouch! Let's do something else," Thea says. The girls decide to make Spoon Bells. They each take a yard-long string, tie a large spoon in the middle, wrap the string ends around their index fingers, and bring them to their ears. They lean forward and tap the dangling spoons on the kitchen counter, tables, and chairs. A gentle tap sends vibrations up the string to Thea's ears. Gong! Just like a church bell!	Kaneesha and her friend Thea cannot agree about the TV volume. Thea likes it low, and Kaneesha likes it loud enough to feel the vibrations through her chair. Instead of arguing, the girls make Spoon Bells and walk around the kitchen, banging their spoons against the counters and furniture. Kaneesha pulls out an oven rack and hits her spoon on it forcefully to get a big bang. Wow! She scrapes the spoon across the rungs. She likes the metallic reverberations. The racket is music to her ears.

Auditory Discrimination—"Huh?"

The child may have difficulty detecting likenesses and differences in words. She may find it hard to pick out or attend to the teacher's voice without being distracted by background noises. Her receptive language may suffer: She may be a poor listener and struggle to read. She may seem noncompliant or may not follow directions well, because she cannot decode what was said. Her expressive language may be inadequate: She may have difficulty participating in conversations, answering questions, and putting her thoughts into writing.

HOW AUDITORY DISCRIMINATION
AFFECTS A CHILD'S BEHAVIOR

A Typical Child	A Child with Poor Auditory Discrimination
Aleah's preschool teacher sings, "This old man, he played two, he played knick-knack on my . . ." She pauses and leans forward, inviting her four-year-old students to fill in the rhyme. Someone says, "Shoe!" Aleah says, "No, not shoe this time. Goo!" The teacher and most of the children laugh. "Goo" rhymes with "two," so it meets the criterion, and it certainly is silly!	"This old man, he played four, he played knick-knack on my. . . ." The teacher leans toward Leslie and invites her to supply a rhyming word. "Five!" Leslie says. "Tell me a word that sounds like 'four,'" the teacher says. "Six!" Leslie says. Her difficulty with auditory discrimination and cohesion means she neither understands the task nor the joke. She just doesn't get it.

A phenomenon often observed is that a child who ordinarily does not talk much or well will begin to speak once she gets moving. Indeed, when she runs or swings, she may suddenly shout, sing, or talk. As self-therapy, to start verbalizing her thoughts, she may jump up to walk around the room. Active movement primes the pump, and speech begins to flow.

The child with vestibular and language problems benefits greatly from therapy that simultaneously addresses both types of dysfunction. Speech-and-language therapists report that just putting the child in a swing during treatment can have remarkable results. Occupational therapists have found that when they treat a child for vestibular dysfunction, speech-and-language skills can improve along with balance, movement, and motor-planning skills. Other treatments include auditory therapy, such as Guy Berard's auditory integration training (AIT), or the method developed by Alfred Tomatis that improves the rhythm of movement and of language. (See p. 338) Some improvements children experience with auditory training include:

- Attention span and focus
- Social interactions
- Speech and motor control
- Auditory discrimination and sensitivity
- Musical expression
- Self-esteem, mood, and motivation
- Understanding spoken language
- Reading, spelling, and handwriting
- Bilateral coordination
- Physical balance and posture

Other ways to help the schoolchild with auditory dysfunction include softening the sound in a noisy classroom, perhaps with a carpet; placing the child in a spot as far from bubbling fish tanks and doorways as possible; and using visual cues to help him supplement auditory information he may miss.

Determining the cause of a child's hearing difficulties is important in order to treat it appropriately. When SPD is the root, a speech/language pathologist or an occupational therapist trained to provide sensory integration therapy is the logical choice. When SPD is not the cause of hearing problems, professionals who provide advice and treatment might include a pediatrician, an otologist (a medical doctor specializing in ear diseases) or an audiologist (a specialist in evaluating hearing disabilities).

HOW MOVEMENT
AFFECTS A CHILD'S AUDITORY FUNCTION

A Typical Child	A Child with Auditory Dysfunction
The fourth-graders can't go outside for recess because it's raining, so Hayley chatters with her friends as they work on a jigsaw puzzle. When math begins after recess, the kids can't settle down. The teacher begins class with the "Hokey Pokey." Shaking her arms, legs, and head, and turning herself about, Hayley begins to feel alert again. When the teacher asks her for the answer to a math problem, Hayley responds correctly.	Caitlin misses recess on rainy days. Restless, she wanders around the room. The "Hokey Pokey" doesn't help, as she can't understand the directions. She feels sleepy when math begins. The teacher asks her an easy question. She can't answer. The next day is sunny, and the kids go out. Caitlin swings the whole time. Later, the teacher asks her to answer another math problem. Caitlin gets it right. The teacher wonders why Caitlin is sometimes "on" and sometimes "off."

CHARACTERISTICS OF AUDITORY
DYSFUNCTION

These checklists will help you gauge whether your child has auditory dysfunction. As you check recognizable characteristics, you will begin to see emerging patterns that help to explain your child's out-of-sync behavior.

The child with difficulty **modulating auditory sensations** may:

☐ Be distressed by loud noises, including the sound of voices.

☐ Be distressed by sudden noises, such as thunder, fire alarms, sirens, and balloons popping.

☐ Be distressed by tinny or metallic sounds, such as those coming from a xylophone or from clinking silverware.

☐ Be distressed by high-pitched sounds, such as those coming from whistles, violins, sopranos, and screeching chalk.

☐ Be distressed by sounds that do not bother others, such as a toilet flushing, a distant church bell, or soft background music.

With poor **auditory discrimination,** the child may:

☐ Seem unaware of the source of sounds or may look all around to locate where they come from.

☐ Have difficulty recognizing particular sounds, such as voices or cars coming down the street.

☐ Have difficulty tracking a sound in the environment, such as footsteps.

☐ Have difficulty recalling, repeating, and referring to words, phrases, conversations, song lyrics, or instructions, both right away (immediate memory) and later (deferred memory).

☐ Have difficulty recognizing the difference between sounds, such as near or distant banging, angry or pleasant voices, or high or low notes.

☐ Be unable to focus or maintain attention to a voice, conversation, story, or sound without being distracted by other sounds.

☐ Have difficulty associating new sounds to familiar sounds, or visual symbols (letters, numerals, musical notes) to their particular sounds.

☐ Have difficulty hearing or reading jokes, verbal math problems, crossword puzzle definitions, or discussions, and understanding how all the information fits together into a coherent whole.

☐ Have a poor sense of timing and rhythm when clapping, marching, singing, jumping rope, or playing rhythm band instruments.

The child may also have difficulty with **receptive language**, and may:

☐ Have a problem discriminating similar sounding word sounds, especially consonants at ends of words, as in cap/cat, bad/bag, side/sign.

☐ Have a short attention span for listening to stories or for reading.

☐ Misinterpret questions and requests.

☐ Be able to follow only one or two instructions in sequence.

☐ Look to others before responding.

☐ Frequently ask for repetition, or be less likely than others to ask for clarification of ambiguous directions or descriptions.

☐ Have difficulty recognizing rhymes.

☐ Have difficulty learning new languages.

The child may have difficulty with **expressive language**, and may:

☐ Have been a late talker.

☐ Have difficulty putting thoughts into spoken or written words.

☐ Talk "off topic," e.g., talk about her new shirt when others are discussing zoo animals or a soccer game.

☐ Have difficulty "closing circles of communication," i.e., responding to others' questions and comments on demand.

☐ Have difficulty correcting or revising what she has said so that others can understand.

☐ Have a weak vocabulary.

☐ Use immature sentence structure (poor grammar and syntax).

☐ Have poor spelling skills.

☐ Have a limited imagination in fantasy play.

☐ Have difficulty making up rhymes.

☐ Sing out of tune.

☐ Have difficulty with reading, especially out loud.

☐ Require more time than other children to respond to sounds and voices.

The child may have difficulty with **speech and articulation,** and may:

☐ Be unable to speak clearly enough to be understood.

☐ Have a flat, monotonous voice quality.

☐ Speak very loudly or very softly.

☐ Speak with a hoarse, husky, strident, weak, or breathy voice.

☐ Speak hesitantly or without fluency and rhythm.

In general, the child may:

☐ Be tired at the end of the day.

☐ Have little motivation or interest in school work.

☐ Have difficulty planning tasks and getting organized.

☐ Be awkward and uncoordinated in movement.

☐ Have poor timing and poor athletic skills.

☐ Have low self-esteem.

☐ Be shy and tend to withdraw from social scenes.

☐ Improve the ability to speak while or after experiencing intense movement.

Part II of this book will give you specific, practical advice as you begin the process of evaluation, diagnosis, and treatment. You will also find many suggestions and activities to help your child at home and at school.

Part II

Coping with

Sensory

Processing

Disorder

Chapter Eight

DIAGNOSIS AND TREATMENT

This chapter will help you learn to recognize and document your child's out-of-sync behavior. It suggests when and how to seek a professional evaluation and diagnosis. It includes descriptions of various kinds of intervention, with emphasis on OT/SI, which is occupational therapy (OT) using a sensory integration (SI) framework.

A PARENT'S SEARCH FOR ANSWERS

A mother wrote me this letter:

"By the time Rob was two, I felt he had a special need, but I couldn't figure out what it was. He required constant attention. Time-outs didn't work because I couldn't contain him. He was defiant, disobedient, disrespectful, and demanding. He was always busy, always talking (great verbal skills!), strong willed, contrary, and easily frustrated. I felt blessed to have Rob, and wouldn't trade him for the world, of course, but he constantly tested and rejected me.

"What was the reason for his behavior? How could I regain control? What method of discipline would get through to him? If his behavior was an attempt to get my attention, how could I supply it in a way that would satisfy him? How could I help a high-energy child channel his energy in a positive direction? I was desperate for answers.

"I started seeking information from my pediatrician. He recommended a neurologist who tested Rob for seizures (he tested normal) and who didn't think he had ADD. Next we saw a psychologist who said Rob was a normal, active, little boy. Then we tried an allergist because he craves milk, and then an ear-nose-throat doctor (ENT) because he seems tired a lot and snores. I thought he might have infected adenoids, but he doesn't.

"Then we saw a child-development specialist who knew something about sensory problems. He didn't do a formal evaluation but could tell that Rob has an immature, underreactive vestibular system with delays in auditory and visual processing. He gave us specific suggestions for activities to do at home, but they didn't work well because Rob didn't cooperate. Since home therapy wasn't working, we then tested Rob for ADD (negative).

"Finally, a neighbor gave me the name of an OT who did a formal evaluation. At three and a half, he was diagnosed with Sensory Processing Disorder. It was a double relief to have Rob's problem identified and to learn that therapy really helps! After four sessions with her, she feels that with a few months of therapy, Rob has good potential to benefit from OT and that his 'nerve problem' will be repaired, and then managing his behavior will be easier.

"The pediatrician feels the therapy won't change anything and suggests using more discipline and seeing a child psychologist. But we have already begun to see results and want to continue the occupational therapy for as long as the OT feels it is necessary. I am hoping we are on the right track.

"This is so unlike anything I have ever been through. This is so hard for me. I am a very 'up' person with lots of friends who call me for advice, and for the first time in my adult life I need advice, big time! I've always worked hard to make our lives 'perfect,' but just getting through the day with Rob has been an accomplishment.

"We're not done yet, but we're making progress. Instead of feeling all alone and desperate, now I'm excited and hopeful. When I see Rob's sweet, loving nature emerging, I feel certain we'll restore harmony in our home."

RECOGNIZING WHEN YOUR CHILD
NEEDS PROFESSIONAL HELP

Ordinarily, growing older means that a child builds upon skills already acquired. A typical child develops the capacity to run after learning to walk, after learning to stand, after learning to creep.

For the out-of-sync child, however, growing older does not always mean getting better at many physical and intellectual tasks, because the basic foundation for efficiently organizing sensory information isn't solid enough.

If growing older doesn't help, what does? Early intervention! The most appropriate intervention for Sensory Processing Disorder is OT/SI, which helps the child develop his nervous system.

Before receiving OT/SI or any other form of intervention, the child will need a professional evaluation and a diagnosis. How do you know if an evaluation is necessary?

Seven Rationalizations That Prevent
Recognizing SPD

At least seven rationalizations prevent some people from recognizing SPD and thus seeking a diagnosis. Educators and therapists often hear these comments.

1) *"Looks like ADHD, sounds like ADHD, must be ADHD."* Symptoms of SPD may look like symptoms of several other problems.

2) *"Never heard of it, so it can't be important."* Many pediatricians, teachers, and other early childhood experts are unfamiliar with SPD and unable to explain it to parents. Fortunately, it is beginning to be widely acknowledged as more research studies and books in layman's terms reach the general public.

3) *"Not my kid!"* Even when parents do learn something about SPD, they may be reluctant to believe that it affects their child. People don't go looking for answers if they are in denial that a problem exists.

4) *"So what if he's not a rocket scientist? We love him just the way he is."* Accepting a child "where he's at" is great, but sometimes parents are too accepting. They may be satisfied with their child's irregular development, even if their child is not.

5) *"So what if she doesn't do what other kids do? She's advanced for her age."* Parents may think their child's unchildlike behavior signifies that she's "too smart" for playdough and playgrounds. However, every child needs to be able to play before she is able to succeed at school. The ability to read at the age of five doesn't guarantee that she has the physical, social, and emotional readiness for kindergarten.

What looks like precocious behavior may, in fact, indicate neurological dysfunction. Johnny pulled himself to a stand in his crib at five months. At nine months, he walked—on tiptoes! His parents thought he was way ahead of other babies until they learned that his tactile defensiveness drove him to avoid touching the crib sheet and the ground.

The child may skip typical childhood experiences because she can't do them. It's illuminating to ask oneself what she avoids. The answer may be elusive, for parents may not realize how much moving, touching, and playing matter. This is a common scenario among families in which the child is the oldest or only one. Without another, more organized child to compare with the disorganized one, parents may be unfamiliar with age-appropriate skills.

6) *"He's so smart, so what if he can't tie his shoes?"* Despite having SPD, the child may have many strengths. He may be a math whiz, a dinosaur expert, or a great storyteller. By contrast, the same child may be weak in self-help skills, sports, or handwriting.

Often, the out-of-sync child develops one or two "splinter skills." These are skills that the child works exceedingly hard to master, but they don't help him generalize his learning to accomplish more complex skills.

For example, one of my preschool students learned to play "Frère Jacques" on the xylophone. He was pleased as punch. Unfortunately, that was his only tune. He played it repeatedly and could not be persuaded to try "Old MacDonald," another simple tune. Another child learned to ride a small bicycle at school—a great accomplishment. However, she had no concept of how to apply her skills to a slightly larger bike at home.

When the child is adept in several areas, or achieves a splinter skill, parents, teachers, and pediatricians frequently believe that she has no definable problems. They think she's "just lazy" about learning new skills.

7) *"He can do everything well, if he wants to."* The child may have good days, when he's cooperative, calm, and competent, and bad days, when he's furious, fidgety, and frustrated. Because SPD can manifest itself in different ways, at different times, it is easy to be lulled into false confidence that dysfunction is not the problem.

Parents may believe that the child's erratic behavior is a matter of choice. It isn't. No child chooses to be disorganized, but the out-of-sync child may be chronically inconsistent in behavior.

Three Valid Reasons to Seek Help

Still uncertain whether to seek a diagnosis? If so, consider the following criteria.

1) *Does the problem get in the child's way?* The answer is yes if he struggles with "doing what comes naturally": creeping, running, jumping, climbing, talking, listening, hugging, and playing. The answer is also yes if he has low self-esteem. Indeed, low self-esteem is a red flag of SPD. Sometimes the child will be referred to a mental health professional. But, if the underlying neurological problems are not addressed, the child develops only compensatory techniques, at most.

2) *Does the child's problem get in other people's way?* Yes, if it causes behavior that may not bother the child but bothers everyone else. The child may annoy other children when he pushes, may vex his teacher when he fidgets, and may scare the bejeepers out of his parents when he's reckless—without comprehending why they are always upset with him.

Yes, if the child is an "angel at home," where it's safe, but a "devil on the street," where it's unpredictable and scary. Yes, if he's an angel at school, where he manages to pull himself together, but a demon at home, where he falls apart at the end of the day. When his behavior differs dramatically in different situations, he is sending out signals of distress.

3) *Should you listen when a teacher, pediatrician, or friend suggests you seek help?* Yes, if they have dealt with many children and can recognize disorganized behavior. While their advice may hurt, it may also confirm what you sense but have been unable to address. Think of it this way: If the gas station attendant says your car needs a tune-up because it isn't functioning well, you would listen. How about a tune-up for your out-of-sync child?

DOCUMENTING YOUR CHILD'S BEHAVIOR

Parents know their child best but often can't make sense of what they know. Perhaps you're concerned about your child's difficulties, which don't fit into traditional medical categories of children's illnesses or disabilities. Perhaps the pediatrician can't identify the problem, either, and says, "Nothing is wrong. Everything will eventually turn out all right."

What should you do?

First, trust your instincts, and then document your observations.

Documentation is a critical part of the process of identifying and addressing your child's needs. Anecdotal evidence is just as important as professional diagnosis. Jot down observations you have made at home and incidents teachers have noted at school. Then, armed with specific data, you will be better equipped to notice patterns and to describe your child's difficulties to a doctor or therapist who is familiar with SPD.

Remember Tommy, Vicki, and Paul? (See pp. 4–7.) Tommy's problems are tactile; Vicki's are vestibular; Paul's are proprioceptive. (These imaginary children have obvious problems. In real life, dysfunction is not so clear-cut.)

Below are charts that their parents prepared. The first chart for each child documents the "hard times": situations that cause out-of-sync behavior. The second chart documents the "easy times": situations in which Tommy, Vicki, and Paul function well. (Charts for Sebastian, the overactive and awkward sensory craver, would be similar.)

You may wish to make charts, too, and fill them with clues to help you solve the mystery of your beautiful, but bewildering, child.

Tommy's Troubling Times
(Tactile Dysfunction)

Because no one seems able to help, Tommy's parents decide to do some detective work. They begin to chart his most difficult moments, hoping to discover patterns that will offer clues about his behavior. Here is their chart:

Behavior	Date Time	Circumstances
Tantrum! Refused to get dressed.	Oct. 10 8:30 am	Says his socks are too tight and he hates his new turtleneck sweater.
Inconsolable at school.	Oct. 14 10:00 am	Teacher said he was fine until it was time for art project (finger painting).
Threw plate on kitchen floor.	Oct. 22 Noon	I thought he'd like cheddar cheese (instead of yogurt) for a change. Wrong!
Screamed in grocery store. Threw a grape at friendly old lady.	Nov. 23 4:30 pm	Day before Thanksgiving. Noisy, crowded store. Old lady (stranger) tousled his hair.
Single-handedly destroyed toys at "Santa's Workshop."	Dec. 18 2:00 pm	Excited by toys in the department store and couldn't keep his hands off them. Out of control, like a bull in a china shop.

INTERPRETATION OF TOMMY'S TROUBLING TIMES

Unrelated as the charted notations seem, they indicate a pattern of tactile dysfunction. Let's look at the incidents, one by one.

First incident: Tommy fusses over his clothes because he is uncomfortable in high collars and bumpy socks. He is not purposely ornery. He simply cannot explain why certain textures are irritating. His poorly regulated tactile system is the culprit, telling him on a subconscious level that his clothes are threatening his sense of well-being. His mother remarks, "The person who invents the truly seamless sock will make a fortune!"

Second incident: Tommy is inconsolable at school, because of finger painting. The teacher, believing that she offers pleasurable activities to her students, is mystified and urges Tommy to participate.

He hates the thought of wet, messy hands, feels like a failure, and wishes the teacher would leave him alone. The scene escalates into a very unhappy situation.

Third incident: Tommy makes a scene at lunch. He has eating problems, for his mouth is overly sensitive to the food textures. If you remember the first time you put a raw oyster in your mouth, you can sympathize! Tommy will eat yogurt because it is familiar and safe. Lumpy cottage cheese, however, is not safe. Tommy can't explain that his defensive tactile system is sending up alert signals, so he hurls down his plate.

Fourth incident: In the supermarket, Tommy bops a friendly woman on the head with a grape. Why does he lash out, making his mother wish she could just abandon him and the Thanksgiving turkey and go home to weep? The answer is simple: To Tommy, the woman is a threat. She is unfamiliar, and she makes the "mistake" of patting him on the head.

For all of us, our heads are extra sensitive to unexpected, light touch. Most of us react instantly to light touch in order to protect the body parts we need for survival. Because Tommy is more sensitive than most, he reacts with what we might consider an excessive response.

Fifth incident: Tommy tears into the toys at Santa's Workshop. Whereas others his age may be satisfied to look at and maybe caress the toys, with a discriminative touch, Tommy "attacks" them. An aspect of his out-of-sync touch system requires him to manhandle objects in order to learn about them. Poor Tommy! He wreaks havoc in Santa's Workshop because he wants to know (and, of course, own) all the toys.

In summary, Tommy has tactile dysfunction, involving over-responsivity and poor discrimination.

Tommy's Terrific Times

Noting Tommy's out-of-sync behavior gives only half the picture. Tommy's parents also chart his terrific times, when he is more positively in sync.

Behavior	Date Time	Circumstances
Fell asleep easily.	Oct. 11 7:30 pm	Asked for a backrub: "Daddy do it, not Mommy." (Art was pleased; usually Tommy prefers me to his Dad.) "Down, not up!" Art rubbed his back hard with firm, downward strokes and gave ten tight bear hugs for more deep pressure. Then Tommy asked Art to put him to bed—a first!
Enjoyed bath and again fell asleep easily.	Oct. 12 7:30 pm	Two good ideas: having Tommy help get the water temperature "just right" (lukewarm), and using Art's rubbing technique, first with a washcloth, then with a sponge. "More, Mommy, more!" The rubbing relaxed him.
Had a great day at school.	Oct. 15 9:00 am– Noon	After I told his teacher that he likes rubdowns, she tried the "People Sandwich" game. He was the "baloney," squished between two gym mats. Loved it. Rest of the day went well.
Ate lunch without complaint.	Oct. 15 12:30 pm	Gave him pureed soup—no lumps. He chowed it down and had a second bowl. Why did it take me so long to realize he'll eat only smooth food?
Actually enjoyed trip to grocery store.	Nov. 30 3:00 pm	Went to supermarket that has miniature carts for kids. He liked pushing one, loaded with potatoes and apples, and was a great helper. Good idea to take him when store isn't crowded.

Behavior	Date Time	Circumstances
Sat on kitchen floor and kept me company for an hour while I baked.	Jan. 5 2:00 pm	His teacher said he enjoyed handling dried beans in the big bin. (He avoids the bin when it has water or sand.) I filled a dishpan with peas, pinto beans, and lentils and gave him some measuring cups and a scoop. He busily measured and poured beans, chatting away. He said, "This is fun work."

INTERPRETATION OF TOMMY'S
TERRIFIC TIMES

First incident: Firm, predictable touch has always comforted Tommy. He asks for a back rub with downward strokes—the way hair grows. (Upward strokes "ruffle his feathers" and "rub him the wrong way.") He prefers his father's deep pressure to his mother's gentler caresses. Firm, soothing pressure suppresses his overresponsivity and prepares him for sleep.

Second incident: Tommy's mother invites him to help adjust the water temperature before he gets in the bath. He likes having some control, rather than being plunged into water that is "too hot!" or "too cold!" Tonight, he climbs in willingly. Also, she takes a cue from her husband and rubs Tommy's back and limbs firmly with a washcloth and sponge, instead of sprinkling him clean. He relaxes, and the result is another pleasant bedtime.

Third incident: The teacher tries a deep-pressure activity at school, with much success. Tommy enjoys being pounded with "mustard" and crawled over by his classmates. Therapeutic and fun, the "People Sandwich" activity also helps him interact with his peers.

Fourth incident: Tommy cannot tolerate lumps in his food. When his mother prepares soup with a smooth texture, he likes it.

Fifth incident: Tommy likes pushing the little grocery cart. He can get a good grip on the smooth handlebar, which doesn't irritate his hands. The deep muscle work of pushing something with resistance feels good. Also, Tommy's mother is paying more attention to his fear of crowds. She notes that going to the store when it is quiet makes the outing enjoyable.

Sixth incident: Tommy likes handling the dried beans because they aren't sticky, and he becomes engrossed in his play. Comparing notes about his behavior, his mother and teacher can strategize ways to provide him with successful tactile experiences at home and school.

Vicki's Vicissitudes (Vestibular Dysfunction)

Vicki's parents take notes about their child's inconsistent behavior:

Behavior	Date Time	Circumstances
Strolling to corner mailbox, stumbled and fell. Cried, "So tired. Carry me!"	June 4 9:30 am	After a long night's sleep and good breakfast, why should she be so limp? But sometimes, by the end of the day, she's raring to go!
Refused to let me leave her at Ellen's birthday party. Once the games began, she became wound up and uncontrollable.	June 9 2:30 pm	So excited about the party, until we arrived. The whole class was invited to play tag and relay races. I was the only mom who had to stay, and Vicki was the only child who didn't play. When she finally left my side, the activities really wound her up. She was in everybody's face, shouting, pushing, and running wildly. Everyone was in tears. We left early.

Behavior	Date Time	Circumstances
Fell apart at the playground. Tantrum lasted twenty minutes.	July 3 2:30 pm	Yesterday she loved the playground; today she hated it. Same place, same time, same weather, but different child! All I did was spin her a few times on the tire swing. Usually, she loves the tire swing.
When we pointed to the moon, she kept looking at our fingers rather than the sky.	Sept. 4 9:30 pm	Up later than usual. Other kids at neighborhood picnic excited about the bright moon and stars. Vicki didn't understand what she was supposed to be looking at.

INTERPRETATION OF VICKI'S VICISSITUDES

First incident: Vicki's early-morning fatigue is a symptom of low muscle tone; she has a loose and limp body. A short excursion to the corner mailbox requires more energy than she can muster at the moment. Also, her trunk is unstable, and she has poor postural responses, poor balance, and poor motor coordination. Her mother notes, however, that in the evening, Vicki is energetic after experiencing intense movement.

Second incident: New situations distress Vicki. Difficulty controlling her movements causes her to be emotionally insecure, so she clings to her mother. Poor coordination and poor motor planning hinder her ability to socialize effectively with her classmates. Her need for vigorous movement is keen, but when she eventually joins in the games, she goes overboard, crashing and bumping into the other children.

Third incident: Knowing that Vicki often enjoys the tire swing, her mother thinks she'll enjoy it even more with a little help to make it spin faster. Vicki cannot tolerate the unexpected, passive movement, however. Vicki hates being on the tire swing when someone else moves it; she likes it only when she is in control.

Fourth incident: Looking at the moon poses another problem. Vicki's eye movements are not well coordinated. Because her eyes don't work well together, she has poor eye-teaming and poor depth perception. She looks at her parents' wagging fingers, within her visual range, and seems unable to gaze beyond her immediate space.

In summary, Vicki is underresponsive to vestibular sensations. Associated problems are low muscle tone, dyspraxia and postural dysfunction, and poor ocular control.

Vicki's Victories

Vicki's parents also take notes about successful situations.

INTERPRETATION OF VICKI'S VICTORIES

First incident: Positioning herself upside down, feet in the air, is a form of self-therapy. Although this position seems odd, it helps regulate Vicki's inefficient processing. Through her inner ear she is receiving useful information about the pull of gravity.

Second incident: Vicki enjoys swinging in different ways for an unusually long time. When she decides how to move and for how long, she is actively engaging in self-therapy. Hanging upside down provides one kind of intense vestibular intake that her brain craves. Swaying gently back and forth, a form of linear movement through space, is soothing. Spinning on the tire swing, a form of rotary movement, also helps regulate her vestibular system.

The fact that she does not get dizzy when she spins indicates that her vestibular system is out of sync. Normally, prolonged spinning would make a person feel woozy, but it makes Vicki feel wonderful.

After swinging, she is chatty and vivacious. The activities have aroused the language centers of her brain. Like all children, she has a lot to say; unlike most children, she often has trouble getting the words out. When she "primes the pump," the words begin to flow.

Third incident: Rocking from side to side is a form of linear motion called oscillation. Like swinging, it organizes Vicki's

Behavior	Date Time	Circumstances
Spent 5 minutes standing on her head. Afterwards, was calm and attentive.	June 6 8:00 pm	Tried to get Vicki into bed to listen to a story, but she was revved up, walking in circles. Finally, she went to the corner and got into an upside-down position. I read the story and she listened quietly. Then she came back to earth, climbed into bed, and fell instantly asleep.
At park, swung for forty-five minutes! Bubbly, bright, and talkative all afternoon.	July 2 2:30 pm	First, she lay across the swing, tummy down, and pushed with her toes. Second, she sat on the swing and asked me to push her for a very long time. Third, she spun herself around on the tire swing. She wasn't dizzy, but I was, just watching!
Tipped to and fro on a makeshift teeter-totter. Later, seemed more in sync than usual.	July 12 2:30 pm.	Vicki joined other kids as they played on a teeter-totter they had made with a plywood board over railroad timber. She rocked from side to side and enjoyed the jolt whenever the edge of the board hit the ground. She had a lot of fun coming up with different ways to balance.
Played happily (for a change!) with other kids at the lake.	Aug. 1 4:00 pm	Instead of throwing and catching the ball, she had fun sitting and lying on it. When she fell off onto the grass, she laughed. The other kids were interested in her ideas, and they all took turns. It's great to see her playing with others!

vestibular system. She likes the jolting sensation when the board strikes the ground. The jolts arouse her in a positive way by sending extra messages to her joints and muscles. When she directs her own play, she plays with purpose and with good attention.

Fourth incident: Tossing a beach ball is too great a challenge, due to Vicki's poor motor skills. However, she enjoys a different challenge: maintaining her balance while sitting on the ball. Every child has an inner drive to resist gravity. Sometimes all the child needs is the right equipment in the right place at the right time! When the other children join her game, Vicki's self-confidence soars, and she is able to play with them happily.

Paul's Problems (Proprioceptive Dysfunction)

Paul's parents prepare this chart as they look for patterns:

Behavior	Date Time	Circumstances
Walked into a telephone pole and required three stitches.	July 9 3:30 pm	Leaving ice cream parlor, he was paying attention to his cone, not to where he was going. So exasperating and frustrating!
Picked up Granny's china figurine; then, smashed it to smithereens when he set it down.	Aug. 2 8:00 pm	Maybe he was tired after long trip getting to Granny's, but even when he's rested he's clumsy. Granny's unhappiness worsened the situation. She wasn't angry at him, just sad; he was inconsolable.
Trying to play catch with a beach ball, he missed it every time.	Aug. 4 Noon	Paul either lunges at the ball at the wrong time or swats it away. His younger cousins are so mean and say, "Baby! Baby! Don't you even know how to catch a ball?"

Behavior	Date Time	Circumstances
At the restaurant, spilled his milk on the tablecloth and his good clothes.	Labor Day 6:30 pm	Sometimes Paul can't seem to manage getting milk into his mouth. Even though the waitress was a sweetheart, Paul was distraught.
Late for first day of fourth grade because he had a fit buttoning his new shirt.	Sept 6 8:30 to 9:30 am	First he resisted wearing the shirt, and then buttoned it incorrectly, saying, "They made it wrong. I never do anything right." He works so hard to do the simplest things.

INTERPRETATION OF PAUL'S PROBLEMS

First incident: Paul bumps into a pole because eating the cone requires his full attention. He really can't chew and walk at the same time. His mother's frustration is nothing compared to Paul's!

Second incident: Paul misjudges the weight of Granny's figurine. Of course, Granny is upset. It's hard to understand that poor control over the force he puts into every movement causes his carelessness.

Third incident: It's about as easy for Paul to catch a beach ball as it is for most of us to capture a butterfly. He has trouble moving through space, coordinating his arms and legs, and anticipating the impact of the ball. No wonder his cousins are "so mean!" They don't like to play with him because they can't predict what he will do and how he will do it. They notice his jerky movements and consider him a "jerk."

Fourth incident: The outing to a restaurant is a disaster. When Paul picks up a glass that feels unfamiliar, the sensations from his muscles can't tell him how much effort to exert. The glass of milk flies through the air, and Paul, once again, makes a mess.

Fifth incident: Buttoning a stiff shirt is hard for Paul. Normal first-day-of-school anxiety, plus Mother's urgings to move faster, plus his clumsiness, add up to Paul's deep despair. Because he moves inefficiently, he has low self-esteem. When he cries, "I never do anything right," he really believes what he says.

In summary, Paul's main problem is poor discrimination of proprioceptive, tactile, and vestibular sensations, along with sensory-based motor disorder.

Paul's Positives

Paul's parents also record his positive experiences:

Behavior	Date Time	Circumstances
Pleased to write a brief note to Granny before our trip.	July 28 3:30 pm	Before starting to write, Paul cracked all his knuckles and squeezed his fingers. Explained, "My hands work better when I do this." Wrote without breaking the pencil point!
Loved playing Granny's "Posture Game."	Aug. 4 10:00 am	Granny challenged him to walk around with a cookbook on his head longer than she can. Paul "won" and earned a trip to the baseball card shop. She makes him "shape up." He adores her.
Enjoyed a tug-of-war game on the beach.	Aug. 7 Noon	We had to play a silly game of tug-of-war with cousins to prove that our family is just as strong as theirs. Paul loved it! Said, "It's awesome to be on a team." He's developing a competitive streak this summer. Astonishing.

Behavior	Date Time	Circumstances
Helped wash Ron's car; then volunteered to wash mine, too.	Dec. 28 2:00 pm	Paul volunteered to lug buckets of water from the house. He can lift a really heavy weight! Enjoyed helping Ron sponge and dry the car. He said, "I bet you're glad to have a son like me." It's a joy to hear him say that. We need to assign him more chores.

INTERPRETATION OF PETER'S POSITIVES

First incident: Paul is "waking up" his writing muscles when he cracks his knuckles and squeezes his fingers. He needs extra stimulation in his hands to manipulate a pencil. His mother remarks that after this exercise he doesn't break the pencil point, as usual.

Second incident: Granny's technique to improve Paul's posture is therapeutically sound. The weight of the book compresses the muscles in his neck and shoulders and gives him extra sensory information. He stands up straighter, in an adaptive behavior to resist gravity. Granny's technique is also psychologically sound. She guesses correctly that he will accept her challenge because it is fun and not too demanding. Succeeding boosts his self-esteem, and tomorrow he may try a bigger challenge—like a dictionary!

Third incident: Pulling the rope organizes Paul's proprioceptive system. He enjoys the tug-of-war because stretching his muscles feels good. He also likes being on a team where everyone is working together and no one can be singled out as the "loser." Like all children, Paul has the inner drive to use his muscles effectively, but he is not a "self-starter." He doesn't know how to engage in activities that benefit his proprioceptive system unless the opportunity is literally put into his hands.

Fourth incident: Paul stretches his muscles vigorously when he hoists water buckets, squeezes the sponge, and towels the car. This activity energizes him, and he's ready to wash another car. His mother's plan to give him more chores will help Paul, for every child needs to feel useful.

DIAGNOSING THE PROBLEM

Consider the adage, "When you hear hoofbeats, look for horses, not zebras." Documenting your child's responses will help you locate those "horses," the specific situations causing out-of-sync behavior.

Maybe you can spot the problem clearly. Maybe you can't. What should you do? Where do you start? You have three choices:

1) You could take the "wait-and-see" approach—but please don't! It is not advisable to sit back and wait for your out-of-sync child to catch up, if his dysfunction gets in his way every day. Possibly, with time, he will function better—but probably his life will just get harder. Why take a chance, when getting help now may make a tremendous difference in his coping skills?

2) You could improve your child's "sensory diet." Joining forces with the teacher, you could develop a home-and-school program that will help your child strengthen his skills. (See Chapter Nine.)

3) You could seek specialist(s) who will either screen your child for possible risk factors or do a full Sensory Processing Disorder evaluation. (Screenings and evaluations are described below.) Ask the pediatrician first for a referral to a specialist. If the doctor resists this idea for some reason, try one of the support systems listed below.

Where to Turn for Support

Everything we can learn about our children's development makes us better parents and teachers. Whether you are certain or uncertain that your child has SPD, gathering information about his strengths and weaknesses will affect how you educate, discipline, and even regard him.

To get a screening or evaluation, start with either of these free resources, available under *IDEA 04 (Individuals with Disabilities Education Improvement Act of 2004)*:

- Your local early intervention program if your child is under age three. The child is eligible for referral and screening but is only eligible for evaluation if the screening indicates that a disability is suspected, and then is only eligible for intervention if he or she meets different state requirements.

- Your local school district if your child is three or older. The child may be eligible for an evaluation and suggestions but must meet state eligibility requirements to receive therapy and other services.

Eligibility varies from state to state. Sometimes, eligibility varies from county to county and even from school to school! Therefore, understanding your locale's requirements is very important. This information helps parents have realistic expectations and prevents frustration for parents and schools.

Here's the deal: If your child is eligible, the school is required to provide services. If your child is ineligible, the school is not required to provide services.

A child with a disability is one who meets the criteria for one of thirteen categories including mental retardation, visual, hearing, speech or language impairments, deafness, deafblindness, orthopedic, serious emotional disturbance, autism, traumatic brain injury, or specific learning disabilities and who, because of this disability, requires special education and related services.

SPD may also be considered an "Other Health Impairment," described as "limited strength, vitality or alertness, including a heightened alertness to environmental stimuli that result in limited alertness with respect to the educational environment." This impairment may be due to several problems (one of which is ADHD) that adversely affect the child's educational performance.

IDEA 04 states that a school system is not required to (buy may) take into consideration whether a child has a severe discrepancy between achievement and intellectual ability. In other words, a child who is, say, strong in math and reading but weak in writing and speaking would probably benefit from therapy. But this child may be ineligible if the school does not consider the difference between his strong and weak skills to be wide enough. Regrettably, the child with SPD, whose academic skills are often out of sync with one another, may fall through the cracks because he is "too smart."

If ineligible under IDEA 04, the child with SPD may be eligible under Section 504 of the Rehabilitation Act of 1973, the antidiscrimination law. A child is eligible for accommodations (which may include services) when he has a physical or mental impairment that substantially limits one or more major life activities. Major life activities include functions such as caring for oneself, performing manual tasks, walking, seeing, hearing, speaking, breathing, learning, and working.

If the child is ineligible under both IDEA 04 and Section 504, check with these other places:

- Your child's preschool or early childhood center, which may suggest a few local OTs who are familiar with SI treatment and who work well with children.

- Private, nonprofit mental heath and social service organizations (listed in the telephone directory), which also provide services, often on a sliding scale.

- A multidisciplinary teaching hospital for a full evaluation ("total workup").

- The Occupational Therapy Department of your local children's hospital.

- www.SPDnetwork.org, which posts a free, online directory of local OTs and other experts, and www.devdelay.org, which offers a directory for a small fee.

What Is a Screening?

A screening is a quick and simple procedure during which an OT or other qualified examiner checks whether children have acquired specific skills. Often, groups of children are screened at the same time at schools or early childhood centers.

The purpose of a screening is the early identification of children who may have one or more developmental deficiencies: cognitive, physical, speech and language, psychosocial, self-help, or adaptive.

A screening is a short, informal "look-see." It is neither a test nor an in-depth examination. When it suggests that a child may have a problem, parents are notified and encouraged to have the child fully evaluated.

What Is an Evaluation?

A formal evaluation is a thorough, individualized examination to look at the whole person and measure his or her skills. Depending on the child's problem, the professional would be an occupational therapist, developmental optometrist (eye doctor), audiologist (specialist in problems related to hearing loss), speech/language pathologist, pediatrician, psychologist, special educator and/or social worker. If the child has severe SPD, a multidisciplinary team composed of several of these professionals would provide a more comprehensive report.

One part of the evaluation is a questionnaire that parents complete, such as a medical, sensory-motor, developmental, or family history (see page 41). Sometimes teachers are asked to fill out questionnaires, too. Your answers will help the OT or other professionals assess your child, as patterns of behavior since birth may confirm clinical observations.

Providing information about your child will help you, too. Indeed, after completing a sensory-motor questionnaire, one mother noted, "We've been puzzled by our four-year-old's cautiousness, language delay, picky eating, and sensitivity to touch, but we never understood the connection. Now the pieces are beginning to fit!"

Another part of the evaluation is the child's visit with the OT in a hospital, clinic, office, school, or your home. The evaluation is based on standardized tests and structured observations of your child. Depending on how much testing is required, the evaluation will take from one hour to several hours, spread over several days.

The OT considers the "W" questions: What are the child's strengths and weaknesses? Where, when, how often, and with what intensity do problems occur? What length of time has the child exhibited the problem behavior? What is the age level at which the child performs? What is happening at home or school that may be affecting his ability to function? Who brings out the worst and the best in him? Why, in the OT's opinion, is the child out of sync?

The crucial question is, "What kind of sensory processing problem is this?" Is it tactile defensiveness? Postural, bilateral, or ocular dysfunction? Poor auditory discrimination? Dr. Ayres and her followers have always insisted on determining the child's sensory needs, so that treatment can be specific.

After careful consideration, the therapist writes a detailed report and confers with parents to help them interpret the results. (Sometimes a doctor will make the diagnosis, based on the qualified examiner's report.) Often, the report is informative. If you receive one that is difficult to understand, call the professional back for a better explanation. She wants to help you, not confuse you.

Therapy may not be indicated if a child is simply immature. Abundant sensory-motor experiences over time may be the late bloomer's best treatment. The professional may suggest activities that you can do as a family at home, or that the child's teacher can implement at school. These activities are enjoyable for everybody and help all children strengthen their neurological skills.

If, however, a problem is evident, the professional may recommend direct, individual, therapy sessions. If you decide to enroll your child, you will not be obligated to stick with the professional who conducted the evaluation. Finding the right therapist is important, because a good fit between therapist and child will affect your child's progress.

Who Pays for Treatment?

Although therapy may be clearly indicated for your child, most health insurance policies do not cover the expense. You have a chance of getting coverage if your pediatrician puts into writing that therapy is a medical necessity. However, sensory problems are not always acknowledged as a health problem.

The reason is that Sensory Processing Disorder is not yet included in publications of diagnostic classification systems, such as the *Diagnostic and Statistical Manual* and the *Diagnostic Classification of Mental Health and Developmental Disorders of Infancy and Early Childhood*. When SPD is eventually included, formal recognition of the disorder will support multidisciplinary research and services for children and their families.

Whether or not your child has been identified as being learning disabled, a pronounced problem with educational functioning is sometimes considered to be a sufficient criterion for funding.

If, in addition to SPD, your child has significant medical, physical, and developmental problems, then she is eligible to receive services. If your child is enrolled in a special-education class in a public school, then related services such as occupational therapy, physical therapy, and speech/language therapy are part of the free educational package, if your child qualifies for them.

If a child is eligible under IDEA 2004 or Section 504, the public school district is legally responsible for providing special education and related services and accommodations. If the child is not eligible, parents may still request that teachers and schools provide accommodations for the child, although the teachers and school district are not required to do so.

Otherwise, paying for therapy is up to you.

So—you must weigh the expense versus the benefits.

One benefit is what a therapist offers: her training and expertise, her therapeutic equipment, and her ability to provide experiences that your child can't get elsewhere. Another, most important, benefit is knowing that you are acting in your child's best interest. By investing in treatment now, you forestall problems that may later cause greater pain and more expensive therapy.

You will have many decisions to make, but should you get early intervention for your child, you will probably see an enormous change in his behavior, his feelings, his skills, and your family life.

THE OCCUPATIONAL THERAPIST'S EVALUATION

An occupational therapist will usually evaluate the child in her office. The evaluation is ordinarily a pleasant experience. While costs vary, expect to spend several hundred dollars. This will be money well spent, and it may be covered by health insurance.

Here are some of the areas an OT investigates:

- Fine- and gross-motor developmental levels
- Visual-motor integration (doing puzzles or copying shapes)
- Visual discrimination
- Neuromuscular control (balance and posture)
- Responses to sensory stimulation (tactile, vestibular, and proprioceptive)
- Bilateral coordination
- Praxis (motor planning)

Sensory processing is just one of several issues the OT is qualified to address. She may identify needs in other areas as well, such as attention deficit, language delay, or an auditory, visual, or emotional problem. If she finds that your child has a difficulty different from SPD, or that his needs are greater than her skills can serve, she may refer you to another professional.

Different Therapies, Different Approaches

After an evaluation, the next step is to arrange for treatment. The most beneficial treatment for SPD is occupational therapy using a sensory integration framework (OT/SI).

Occupational Therapy

Occupational therapy (abbreviated as OT) encompasses evaluation, assessment, treatment, and consultation. Occupational therapy is the use of purposeful activity to maximize the independence and the maintenance of health of an individual who is limited by a physical injury or illness, cognitive impairment, a psychosocial dysfunction, a mental illness, a developmental or learning disability, or an adverse environmental condition. For a child, purposeful activities include swinging, climbing, jumping, buttoning, drawing, and writing. Such activities are the child's "occupation."

The specific goals of occupational therapy using a sensory integration (OT/SI) framework are to improve the person's social participation, self-esteem, self-regulation and sensory-motor abilities.

THE OCCUPATIONAL THERAPIST

An occupational therapist (also abbreviated as OT) is a health professional who has received a baccalaureate or master's degree after completing a course of study, plus internship experience, in the biological, physical, medical, and behavioral sciences. (After January 1, 2007, all new OT candidates will require a postbaccalaureate degree.) Coursework includes neurology, anatomy, orthopedics, psychology, and psychiatry.

The OT may work with your child individually or in a group, at school, in a clinic, hospital, community mental health center, or your home. The ideal OT is one who specializes in pediatrics and who has received additional, postgraduate training in sensory integration theory and treatment.

Under the guidance of a therapist, the child actively takes in movement and touch information in playful, meaningful, and natural ways that help his brain modulate these fundamental neural messages. The child responds favorably to SI treatment, because his nervous system is pliable and changeable. Therapy teaches the child to succeed—and he loves it!

ACTIVITIES THE OT MAY PROVIDE

Every child is different, so the sequence and kinds of activity that an occupational therapist provides for your child will be individualized. She will design a program based on his particular needs, going back in his system to where early skills have been mastered. Following his lead, she will guide him through activities that affect his central nervous system and challenge his ability to respond successfully to sensory stimuli in an organized way.

For instance, your child may have difficulty jumping, climbing, pedaling tricycles, and getting dressed. These problems can't be "fixed" by teaching him specifically how to jump, climb, pedal, and put on a jacket, when the underlying problem is SPD. He doesn't need jumping lessons, but opportunities to integrate all sensations. With her appealing equipment and professional knowledge, a qualified therapist can weave art and science together to offer these opportunities.

Here is a small sampling of activities that an OT may provide:

- To reduce tactile defensiveness—having arms and legs rubbed with differently textured sponges and cloths

- To improve tactile discrimination—finding hidden toys by manipulating a ball of therapeutic putty

- To develop better body awareness and improve postural security—swinging prone in a special swing suspended from the ceiling, in order to experience specific movement sensations

- To improve balance—lying or sitting on large, inflated, therapy balls

• To improve bilateral coordination—using a rolling pin with both hands to bat at a ball hanging from the ceiling, while lying prone

• To improve motor planning—moving through obstacle courses

• To improve fine motor skills—playing with magnets to build up the muscles of the hand to stabilize loose joints

• To improve extension against the pull of gravity—riding across the floor, or riding headfirst down a ramp, while lying prone on a scooter

• To improve flexion—clinging to a cylindrical swing that is suspended from the ceiling

• To reduce gravitational insecurity—swinging gently on a flat glider swing; jumping on a bounce pad

• To improve ocular control and visual discrimination—playing games with beanbags, balloons, and suspended balls

The most important factor that will determine the success of therapy is the child's own inner drive to explore and learn from the environment. The child's motivation to spin on a swing, to touch certain textures, or to be gently pressed between two gym mats tells the therapist what the child's nervous system seeks.

According to Dr. Ayres, "Sensations that make a child happy tend to be integrating." When the child is actively involved in his own therapy, he becomes more organized, he has fun, and he feels in sync.

Other Types of Therapy

While the out-of-sync child will benefit most from occupational therapy, sometimes another highly specific type of therapy will also help. (While SPD is a neurological problem, most neurologists are not trained to evaluate it in children, and they do not provide SI therapy.)

PHYSICAL THERAPY

Physical therapy is a health profession devoted to improving an individual's physical abilities. It involves activities that strengthen the child's muscular control and motor coordination, especially of his large muscles. Sometimes using physical agents such as massage, whirlpool baths, or ultrasound, physical therapists help the child get his muscles ready for voluntary movement. Some physical therapists receive additional training in sensory integration theory and treatment. See www.apta.org.

SPEECH-AND-LANGUAGE THERAPY

Speech-and-language therapy includes activities designed to meet specific goals for the child. The child may need help with speech skills, such as pronouncing "L," "K," or "Sh" sounds; monitoring the pitch of his voice; and strengthening oral-motor control in the muscles of his mouth. He may also benefit from activities designed to expand his language skills, such as retelling stories, conversing, and playing games to develop memory and vocabulary. As many children with SPD are picky eaters, therapy with a speech pathologist trained in oral-motor and feeding issues may be very helpful. Indeed, when the child receives cotreatment simultaneously from an occupational therapist who has been trained in this area, optimal benefits of getting in the mouth occur. See www.asha.org.

VISION THERAPY

A developmental optometrist provides a complete evaluation of the visual system, determining not only that a person can see, but also how he sees—the "What is it, Where is it, and Where am I?" functions of vision. After the evaluation, the optometrist will provide the proper lens therapies or vision therapy (VT). VT includes sensory-motor and educational activities that strengthen eye-motor control, visual discrimination, and eye-hand coordination. Along with lenses or prisms, VT helps the child integrate visual information with input from other senses, such as hearing, touching, and moving. This treatment often helps a child's eyes and body function in sync and prevents learning-related visual problems. See www.optometrists.org, www.covd.org, www.pavevision.org, and www.oep.org.

AUDITORY TRAINING

Auditory training is a method of sound stimulation designed to improve a person's listening and communicative skills, learning capabilities, motor coordination, body awareness, and self-esteem. Various methods, including the methods developed by Dr. Alfred Tomatis, Dr. Guy Berard, and Sheila Frick, OTR/L, employ the use of special headphones. During a course of several days, the child listens passively to music and voices filtered through the headphones. Then he participates in active voice work, such as repeating sounds, reading aloud, and conversing. Therapy helps the ear to attend to and discriminate among sounds, the vestibular system to integrate sensory messages of balance and posture, and the person to become more focused, centered, and organized. See www.tomatis.net, or www.VitalLinks.net.

CHIROPRACTIC

Chiropractic is the philosophy, art, and science of detecting and correcting subluxation in the human body. Subluxation is a partial dislocation or abnormal movement of a bone in a joint. Chiropractic helps children with SPD by specifically addressing the structure and function of the nerves, muscles, and joints controlling posture and movement that influence our ability to interact with our environment. See www.chiroweb.com/find/children.html.

CRANIOSACRAL THERAPY

CranioSacral Therapy (CST) is a gentle method of evaluating and enhancing the function of the craniosacral system (the membranes and cerebrospinal fluid that protect the brain and spinal cord). CST involves light-touch manipulation of the bones in the skull, sacrum, and coccyx to correct an imbalance that can adversely affect the development of the brain and spinal cord and can result in sensory, motor, and neurological dysfunction. Developed by Dr. John Upledger, CST is used by a variety of health care professionals. See www.upledger.com.

HIPPOTHERAPY
Hippotherapy means "treatment with the help of the horse." Occupational, physical, and speech therapists use the horse as a modality to improve the posture, movement, neuromotor function, and sensory processing of people with disabilities. The movement of the horse, with traditional therapy intervention, influences muscle tone, encourages muscle action, and improves vestibular reactions, sensory-motor integration, and midline postural control. See www.narha.org or www.nceft.com.

MARTIAL ARTS
For elementary school–aged and older children, martial arts, such as karate and tae kwon do, can be very therapeutic. (Dr. Larry Silver, who wrote the foreword to *The Out-Of-Sync Child,* often recommends martial arts for his clients with SPD.) See www.martialarts.about.com/cs/kids.

NUTRITIONAL THERAPY
Good nutrition is essential for development, efficient maintenance, and functioning, optimum activity level, and resistance to infection and disease. A nutritionist can help a person with nutritional deficiencies achieve balance in carbohydrates, fats, protein, vitamins, minerals, and water. See www.AutismNDI.com.

PERCEPTUAL MOTOR THERAPY
Perceptual motor therapy provides integrated movement experiences that remediate gross-motor, fine-motor, and visual discrimination problems. Activities, including sensory-input techniques, stimulate left/right brain communication to help the child interpret incoming information to the nervous system. Goals are to develop more mature patterns of response to specific stimuli, improve motor skills and balance, and stimulate alternate routes to memory and sequencing for those children who do not respond to the methods taught in the conventional classroom. See www.gmskids.org or www.kidsmovingco.com.

PSYCHOTHERAPY

Psychotherapy is sometimes appropriate, particularly if the child is depressed or has behavior or self-image problems. (Psychotherapy deals with the effects of SPD but not the underlying causes.) Psychotherapies include behavioral therapy, to help the child deal with problematical symptoms and behaviors; family therapy, to help the child, parents, and siblings become a healthier unit; and play therapy, to promote the child's social-emotional development. Therapists include clinical psychologists, licensed clinical social workers, and child psychiatrists. See www.floortime.org.

BRINGING THERAPIST AND CHILD TOGETHER

Before the first session with the OT (or other therapist), you will want to prepare your child. You can say, "Today you'll meet someone who will help you get stronger. She has great toys and games to play. Her place is like a gym where you will do things that feel good. I think you'll have lots of fun."

Emphasizing that therapy will be fun is important. Many children with Sensory Processing Disorder don't have much fun. They wish they could but simply don't know how.

When you think and speak positively about therapy, you help make it work for your child. You reassure your child that this is not punishment or something to feel defensive about. The child may blame himself for being frequently clumsy or tired, saying, "I'm no good." He needs frequent confirmation that he *is* good, and that therapy will make him even better.

Whether treatment takes place in a busy clinic, at school, or in your very own basement, you will be involved, too. Part of the therapist's job is to collaborate with parents to design activities that help the child function better at home. The therapist may also give suggestions to the teacher to modify the classroom environment.

Because treatment will become a part of your child's life, you

225

and your child should get along well with the therapist. Goodness-of-fit is essential! If your child resists going for treatment, or if you lack confidence in the therapist, then something is amiss, and you should switch to another one, if possible. Treatment will be most successful when all the parties have a respectful and pleasant working relationship.

Working with the therapist will take some time and effort, but your involvement is definitely worthwhile. The therapy itself may not last forever, but the results will last a lifetime.

KEEPING A RECORD

If you aren't already keeping a running record of your child's behavior and development, please begin one now! Your record should include:

- Your own documented observations
- Teachers' comments and reports
- Names, addresses, and telephone numbers of professionals you have consulted or intend to consult
- Detailed, dated notes of consultations and telephone conversations with professionals
- Written confirmation of information you have received orally
- Specialists' evaluations, diagnoses, and recommendations

An orderly, chronological notebook is a valuable tool. It will help you see patterns that you may have missed. It will provide evidence of your child's uneven development, should you need to prove at some point that your child requires special services. It will also help you feel more organized and in control.

A professional diagnosis, along with therapy, should bring some relief. Meanwhile, life at home may improve when you follow some of the suggestions offered in the next chapter.

Chapter Nine

YOUR CHILD AT HOME

Parents can make home life easier both for themselves and their child by introducing a balanced "sensory diet," including activities that strengthen neurological development and improve self-help skills.

A PARENT'S REVELATION

When Tonya was three, she entered St. Columba's. Reluctantly. She was fearful and limp. She spoke in a breathy voice, shrank from physical contact, and cried when it was time to go outdoors. However, she was very bright and loved stories, music, and dressing up.

During the fall, we screened the three-year-olds for sensory processing disorder. Tonya's results suggested a possibility of some dysfunction, but we weren't sure. She might have been simply immature.

While we usually observe late bloomers carefully before recommending occupational therapy, we decided to have a conference with Tonya's parents. We felt we could promote Tonya's social and physical development if we could persuade them to improve her sensory diet.

During the conference they listened politely to our suggestions to get Tonya outside every day, to give her more hands-on experiences, and to invite children over to play.

"Well, those ideas won't work," her mother said. "Tonya hates being cold and messy. She dislikes going outside and playing with other kids. She just wants to be with the baby and me and listen to stories." Rising to her feet, she added, "And that's fine with us." Unsatisfactorily for all of us, the conference ended.

And so it went. Since the parents repeatedly resisted our suggestions, we decided to back off.

Then, just as we stepped back, Tonya's little sister took charge at home. This two-year-old began to clamor for changes in the family's lifestyle. Sociable and energetic, she loved playing outside with the neighborhood children. Her mother found that the best way to gratify her was to take her daily to the playground. Of course, Tonya had to go, too.

After Christmas vacation, we noticed a "new" Tonya. She was participating more and playing happily with other children. She laughed, spoke up, and even shouted. Her development amazed and delighted us.

One day, her mother said, "I must tell you, I've had a revelation. We've been going to the park every day, even when it's freezing. Tonya resisted at first, but now she asks to go. You had to tell me over and over again about a sensory diet, until I finally listened. Now I realize that for both girls, a sensory diet makes good sense and a huge difference!"

A BALANCED SENSORY DIET

A balanced sensory diet is a planned and scheduled activity program that a therapist develops to meet the needs of a specific child's nervous system. Its purpose is to help the child become better regulated and more focused, adaptable, and skillful.

The sensory diet concept was developed by occupational therapists Patricia and Julia Wilbarger in the 1990s. One of the best books on the subject is *Building Bridges through Sensory Integration,* by OTs Paula Aquilla, Ellen Yack, and Shirley Sutton (Sensory Resources, 2002).

Just as the main food groups provide daily nutritional requirements, a daily sensory diet fulfills physical and emotional needs. The out-of-sync child needs an individualized diet of tactile, vestibular, and proprioceptive nourishment more than most but doesn't know how to get it. So, we must and can help.

A sensory diet includes a combination of alerting, organizing, and calming activities. An alerting or calming activity may come first, depending on your child's needs.

Alerting activities benefit the underresponsive child, who needs a boost to become effectively aroused. These include:

• Crunching dry cereal, popcorn, chips, crackers, nuts, pretzels, carrots, celery, apples, or ice cubes,

• Taking a shower,

• Bouncing on a therapy ball or beach ball, or

• Jumping up and down on a mattress or trampoline.

Organizing activities help regulate the child's responses. They include:

• Chewing granola bars, fruit bars, licorice, dried apricots, cheese, gum, bagels, or bread crusts,

• Hanging by the hands from a chinning bar,

• Pushing or pulling heavy loads, or

• Getting into an upside-down position.

Calming activities help the child decrease sensory over-responsivity or overstimulation. They include:

• Sucking a pacifier, hard candy, frozen fruit bar, or spoonful of peanut butter,

• Pushing against walls with the hands, shoulders, back, buttocks, and head,

• Rocking, swaying, or swinging slowly to and fro,

• Cuddling or back rubbing, or

• Taking a bath.

When you initiate your own home program for a sensory diet, it is always best to consult a therapist about your child's requirements. What are appropriate activities? Where should your child do them? When? How often? For how long?

Here are some guidelines:

• Set up specific times during the day for a structured sequence (after breakfast, after school, and before bedtime).

• If possible, supply the activity that your child wants. Often, the child will tell you. Even if he can't say, "My nervous system desperately requires an intense movement experience," you may be able to read his mind as he prepares to leap from the playhouse roof. Find another way to let him jump!

• Let the child direct the play. While "more!" may mean more, do supervise so the child doesn't become overaroused. "Stop!" means stop at once. During the activity, watch and listen for nonverbal signals: Relaxation and pleased facial expressions suggest that the activity feels good; whimpers or raucous laughter suggest that it is time to cool down.

• For variety, change the routine and environment.

• Check periodically with the therapist to ensure your home diet is "nutritious" and is meeting your child's varying needs.

A balanced sensory diet is like a fitness plan. It will enhance every child's functioning, whether the child is in or out of sync.

PROMOTING HEALTHY SENSORY PROCESSING AT HOME

Many children seek more touch and movement than others. They are Touchers-and-Feelers, Bumpers-and-Crashers. Their high activity level tells us that if they can play "bumpety bump" on the tire swing, or soar into a leaf pile, or wallow in mud puddles, they will "get it all together." They are right.

Other children avoid touch and movement experiences, which make them uncomfortable. These children need guidance to explore their environment and to feel safe. Once they learn how to play actively, they, too, begin to get it all together.

Following are some ideas for multisensory activities that parents and caregivers can provide for young children at home. Every little body can benefit from these suggestions—not only the children who seek such activities, but also the children who are more tentative about exploring their environment.

Want more? For hundreds of detailed "SAFE" (Sensory-motor, Appropriate, Fun and Easy) activities for children of all ages, see *The Out-of-Sync Child Has Fun* (Perigee, 2003), *101 Activities for Kids in Tight Spaces* (St. Martin's, 1995), and *The Goodenoughs Get in Sync* (Sensory Resources, 2004).

Activities to Develop the Tactile Sense

Rub-a-Dub-Dub—Encourage the child to rub a variety of textures against her skin. Offer different kinds of soap (oatmeal soap, shaving cream, lotion soap) and scrubbers (loofah sponges, thick washcloths, foam pot-scrubbers, plastic brushes).

Water Play—Fill the kitchen sink with sudsy water and unbreakable pitchers and bottles, turkey basters, sponges, eggbeaters, and toy water pumps. Or, fill a washtub with water and toys and set it on the grass. Pouring and measuring are educational and therapeutic, as well as high forms of entertainment.

Water Painting—Give the child a bucket of water and paint-brush to paint the porch steps, the sidewalk, the fence, or her own body. Or, provide a squirt bottle filled with clean water (because the squirts often go in the child's mouth).

Finger Painting—Let the sensory craver wallow in this literally "sensational" activity. Encourage (but don't force) the sensory avoider to stick a finger into the goop. For different tactile experiences, mix sand into the paint, or place a blob of shaving cream, peanut butter, or pudding on a plastic tray. Encourage him to draw shapes, letters, and numbers. If he "messes up," he can erase the error with his hand and begin again.

Finger Drawing—With your finger, "draw" a shape, letter, number, or design on the child's back or hand. Ask the child to guess what it is and then to pass the design on to another person.

Sand Play—In a sandbox, add small toys (cars, trucks, people, and dinosaurs), which the child can rearrange, bury, and rediscover. Instead of sand, use dried beans, rice, pasta, cornmeal, popcorn, and mud. Making mud pies and getting messy are therapeutic, too.

Feelie Box—Cut a hole in a shoebox lid. Place spools, buttons, blocks, coins, marbles, animals, and cars in the box. The child inserts a hand through the hole and tells you what toy she is touching. Or, ask her to reach in and feel for a button or car. Or, show her a toy and ask her to find one in the box that matches. These activities improve the child's ability to discriminate objects without the use of vision.

"Can You Describe It?"—Provide objects with different textures, temperatures, and weights. Ask her to tell you about an object she is touching. (If you can persuade her not to look at it, the game is more challenging.) Is the object round? Cool? Smooth? Soft? Heavy?

Oral-motor Activities—Licking stickers and pasting them down, blowing whistles and kazoos, blowing bubbles, drinking through straws or sports bottles, and chewing gum or rubber tubing may provide oral satisfaction.

Hands-on Cooking—Have the child mix cookie dough, bread dough, or meat loaf in a shallow roasting pan (not a high-sided bowl).

Science Activities—Touching worms and egg yolks, catching fireflies, collecting acorns and chestnuts, planting seeds, and digging in the garden provide interesting tactile experiences.

Handling Pets—What could be more satisfying than stroking a cat, dog or rabbit?

People Sandwich—Have the "salami" or "cheese" (your child) lie facedown on the "bread" (gym mat or couch cushion) with her head extended beyond the edge. With a "spreader" (sponge, pot scrubber, basting or vegetable brush, paintbrush, or washcloth) smear her arms, legs, and torso with pretend mustard, mayonnaise, relish, ketchup, etc. Use firm, downward strokes. Cover the child, from neck to toe, with another piece of "bread" (folded mat or second cushion). Now press firmly on the mat to squish out the excess mustard, so the child feels the deep, soothing pressure. You can even roll or crawl across your child; the mat will distribute your weight. Your child will be in heaven.

Activities to Develop the Vestibular System

Rolling—Encourage your child to roll across the floor and down a grassy hill.

Swinging—Encourage (but never force) the child to swing. Gentle, linear movement is calming. Fast, high swinging in an arc is more stimulating. If the child has gravitational insecurity, start him on a low swing so his feet can touch the ground, or hold him on your lap. Two adults can swing him in a blanket, too.

Spinning—At the playground, let the child spin on the tire swing or merry-go-round. Indoors, offer a swivel chair or Sit 'n Spin. Monitor the spinning, as the child may become easily overstimulated. Don't spin her without her permission!

Sliding—How many ways can a child swoosh down a slide? Sitting up, lying down, frontwards, backwards, holding on to the sides, not holding on, with legs straddling the sides, etc.

Riding Vehicles—Trikes, bikes, and scooters help children improve their balance, motor planning, and motor coordination.

Walking on Unstable Surfaces—A sandy beach, a playground "clatter bridge," a grassy meadow, and a waterbed are examples of shaky ground that require children to adjust their bodies as they move.

Rocking—Provide a rocking chair for your child to get energized, organized, or tranquilized.

Riding, balancing, and walking on a seesaw.

Balancing on a Teeter-Totter—Center a board over a railroad timber. (See *The Out-of-Sync Child Has Fun* for ideas.)

Teeter-Totter:

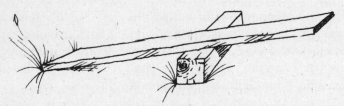

Sitting on a T-stool—A T-stool helps improve balance, posture, and attention. (See *The Out-of-Sync Child Has Fun* for ideas.)

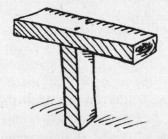

T-Stool:

Balancing on a Large Therapy Ball—Your child can lie on her stomach, on her back, or sit and bounce. Some balls have handles for bouncing up and lower (hippity-hopping).

Tummy Down, Head Up—Have the child lie on her stomach. On the floor, she can rock to and fro to "Row, Row, Row Your Boat"; draw on paper while listening to music, using crayons, which require her to bear down to make a mark; and play with small toys. On a swing or therapy ball, she can "draw" on the ground or carpet with a stick; throw sponges into a basket; and bat a suspended ball with a cardboard tube.

Jogging—Run around the block together!

Activities to Develop the Proprioceptive System

Lifting and Carrying Heavy Loads—Have the child pick up and carry soft-drink bottles to the picnic; laundry baskets upstairs; or grocery bags, filled with nonbreakables, into the house. He can also lug a box of books, a bucket of blocks, or a pail of water from one spot to another.

Pushing and Pulling—Have the child push or drag grocery bags from door to kitchen. Let him push the stroller, vacuum, rake, shove heavy boxes, tow a friend on a sled, or pull a loaded wagon. Hard muscular work jazzes up the muscles.

Hanging by the Arms—Mount a chinning bar in a doorway, or take your child to the park to hang from the monkey bars. When she suspends her weight from her hands, her stretching muscles send sensory messages to her brain. When she shifts from hand to hand as she travels underneath the monkey bars, she is developing upper-body strength.

Hermit Crab—Place a large bag of rice or beans on the child's back and let her move around with a heavy "shell" on her back.

Joint Squeeze—Put one hand on the child's forearm and the other on his upper arm; slowly press toward and away from his elbow. Repeat at his knee and shoulder. Press down on his head. Straighten and bend his fingers, wrists, elbows, knees, ankles, and toes. These extension and flexion techniques provide traction and compression to his joints and are effective when he's stuck in tight spaces, such as church pews, movie theaters, cars, trains, and especially airplanes where the air pressure changes.

Body Squeeze—Sit on the floor behind your child, straddling him with your legs. Put your arms around his knees, draw them toward his chest, and squeeze hard. Holding tight, rock him forward and back.

Bear Hugs—Everyone needs twelve hugs a day.

Pouring—Let the child pour sand, beans, or water from one container to another.

Opening Doors—Is this hard? Then your child needs practice! Take the time to let her do it all by herself.

Back-to-Back Standing Up—Position two children on the floor, back to back. Ask them to "dig their feet into the floor" and to stand up together by pressing against each other's back.

Bulldozer—One child sits in a large cardboard box or on a folded gym mat, and another child pushes the load across the floor, using his head, shoulders, back, or feet to make it move.

Arm Wrestling—If you are stronger than your child, please let him win once in a while.

Activities to Develop the Auditory System

Simplify your language. Speak slowly, shorten your comments, abbreviate instructions, and repeat what you have said. Reinforce verbal messages with gestural communication: facial expressions, hand movements, and body language.

Talk to your child while she dresses, eats, or bathes, to teach her words and concepts, such as nouns (sunglasses, casserole), body parts (thumb, buttocks), prepositions (around, through), adjectives (juicy, soapy), time (yesterday, later), categories (vegetables/fruits), actions (zip, scrub), and emotions (pleased, sorry).

Share your own thoughts. Model good speech and communication skills. Even if the child has trouble responding verbally, she may understand what you say.

Take the time to let your child respond to your words and express his thoughts. Don't interrupt, rush, or pressure him to talk.

Be an active listener. Pay attention. Look your child in the eye when she speaks. Show her that her thoughts interest you.

Help your child communicate more clearly. If you catch one word, say, "Tell me more about the truck." If you can't catch his meaning, have him show you by gesturing.

Reward her comments with smiles, hugs, and verbal praise, such as, "That's a great idea!" Your positive feedback will encourage her to strive to communicate. (Don't say, "Good talking," which means little to the child and implies that all you care about is words, rather than the message the child is trying to get across.)

Use rhythm and beat to improve the child's memory. Give directions or teach facts with a "piggyback song," substituting your words to a familiar tune. Example: To the tune of "Mary Had a Little Lamb," sing, "Now it's time to wash your face, Brush your teeth, comb your hair, Now it's time to put on clothes, So start with underwear!"

Encourage your child to pantomime while listening to stories and poems, or to music without words.

Read to your child every day!

Activities to Develop the Visual System

Making Shapes—Let your child draw or form shapes, letters, and numbers in different materials, such as playdough, finger paint, shaving cream, soap foam, sand, clay, string, pudding, or pizza dough.

Mazes and Dot-to-Dot Activities—Draw mazes on paper, the sidewalk, or the beach. Have the child follow the mazes with his finger, a toy car, a crayon, a marker, or chalk. On graph paper, make dot-to-dot patterns for the child to follow.

Peg Board—Have the child reproduce your design or make his own.

Cutting Activities—Provide paper and scissors and have your child cut fringe and strips. Draw curved lines on the paper for her to cut. Cutting playdough is fun, too.

Tracking Activities—Lie on your backs outside and watch birds or airplanes, just moving your eyes while keeping your heads still.

Jigsaw Puzzles!
Block Building!!

More Activities to Develop Sensory-Motor Skills

Sensory processing is the foundation for fine-motor skills, motor planning, and bilateral coordination. All these skills improve as the child tries the following activities that integrate the sensations.

FINE-MOTOR SKILLS

Flour Sifting—Spread newspaper on the kitchen floor and provide flour, scoop, and sifter. (A turn handle is easier to manipulate than a squeeze handle, but both develop fine-motor muscles in the hands.) Let the child scoop and sift.

Stringing and Lacing—Provide shoelaces, lengths of yarn on plastic needles, or pipe cleaners, and buttons, macaroni, cereal "Os," beads, spools, paper clips, and jingle bells. Making bracelets and necklaces develops eye-hand coordination, tactile discrimination, and bilateral coordination.

Egg Carton Collections—The child may enjoy sorting shells, pinecones, pebbles, nuts, beans, beads, buttons, bottle caps, and other found objects and organizing them in the individual egg compartments.

Household Tools—Picking up cereal pieces with tweezers; stretching rubber bands over a box to make a "guitar"; hanging napkins, doll clothes, and paper towels with clothespins; and smashing egg cartons with a mallet are activities that strengthen many skills.

Office and Classroom Tools—Have the child cut with scissors; use a stapler and hole puncher; draw with crayons and chalk; paint with brushes, feathers, sticks, and eyedroppers; squeeze glue onto paper in letters or designs, sprinkle sparkles on the glue, and shake off the excess; and wrap boxes with brown paper, tape, and string.

MOTOR PLANNING

Jumping from a Table—Place a gym mat beside a low table and encourage the child to jump. After each landing, stick tape on the mat to mark the spot. Encourage the child to jump farther each time.

Walking like Animals—Encourage the child to lumber like a bear, on all fours; a crab, from side to side on all fours; a turtle, creeping; a snake, crawling; an inchworm, by stretching flat and pulling her knees toward her chest; an ostrich, while grasping her ankles; a duck, squatting; a frog, squatting and jumping; a kangaroo or bunny, jumping; a lame dog, with an "injured" leg; a gorilla, bending her knees; a horse, galloping.

Playground Games—Remember Simon Says, Ring-Around-the-Rosy, The Hokey-Pokey, London Bridge, Shoo Fly, and Mother, May I?

Insy-Outsy—Teach the child to get in and out of clothes, the front door, and the car. With a little help, the child may become able to perform these tasks independently, even if it takes a long time!

BILATERAL COORDINATION

Ball Catch—Toss a large beach ball gently to the child from a short distance. As he becomes more competent, use a smaller ball and step farther away.

Ball Whack—Have the child hold a baseball bat, rolling pin, broomstick, book, cardboard tube, or ruler in both hands. Remind her to keep her feet still. Toss her a big ball. As she swings, her body will rotate, as her arms cross the midline.

Two-handed Tetherball—Suspend a sponge ball at the child's eye level from a string attached to a wide doorframe. Let your child choose different "bats." Have her count how many hits she makes without missing. Try four-handed tetherball, in which you play, too.

Balloon Fun—Using both hands together, the child bounces or tosses up a balloon and catches it. He can keep it afloat by whacking it with open hands or batting it repeatedly with hands clasped together in one large "fist."

Rolling-Pin Fun—Provide the child with a cylindrical block or a rolling pin without handles, so he presses down with his opened hands. Have him roll real dough, playdough, crackers, clay—or mud!

Body Rhythms—While you chant or sing, clap, and tap different body parts and have your child imitate your motions. Tip your head from side to side, wave your arms overhead, shake icky sticky glue off your hands, pound your chest, slap your hips, bend from side to side, hunch and relax your shoulders, stamp your feet, and hop from foot to foot. Use both hands together or alternately.

Eggbeater Fun—Give your child an eggbeater to whip up soap-suds or mix up a bowl of birdseed, or of uncooked beans and rice.

Marble Painting—Line a tray or cookie sheet with paper. Put a few dabs of finger paint in the center of the paper. Provide a marble to roll through the paint to make a design. Great wrapping paper!

Ribbon Dancing—Attach ribbons, streamers, or scarves to the ends of a dowel. Holding the dowel with both hands, the child swirls the ribbons overhead, from side to side, and up and down. (No dowel? Give him a ribbon for each hand.) This activity also improves visual-motor coordination.

Two-Sided Activities—Encourage the child to jump rope, swim, bike, hike, row, paddle, and do morning calisthenics.

Suggestions to Develop Self-Help Skills

Self-help skills improve along with sensory processing. The following suggestions may make your child's life easier—and yours, too!

DRESSING

• Buy or make a "dressing board" with a variety of snaps, zippers, buttons and buttonholes, hooks and eyes, buckles and shoelaces.

• Provide things that are not her own clothes for the child to zip, button, and fasten, such as sleeping bags, backpacks, handbags, coin purses, lunch boxes, doll clothes, suitcases, and cosmetic cases.

• Provide alluring dress-up clothes with zippers, buttons, buckles, and snaps. Oversized clothes are easiest to put on and take off.

• Eliminate unnecessary choices in your child's bureau and closet. Clothes that are inappropriate for the season and that jam the drawers are sources of frustration.

• Put large hooks inside closet doors at the child's eye level so he can hang up his own coat and pajamas. (Attach loops to coats and pajamas on the outside so they won't irritate the skin.)

• Supply cellophane bags for the child to slip her feet into before pulling on boots. The cellophane prevents shoes from getting stuck and makes the job much easier.

• Let your child choose what to wear. If she gets overheated easily, let her go outdoors wearing several loose layers rather than a coat. If he complains that new clothes are stiff or scratchy, let him wear soft, worn clothes, even if they're unfashionable.

• Comfort is what matters.

• Set out tomorrow's clothes the night before.

Encourage the child to dress himself. Allow for extra time, and be available to help. If necessary, help him into clothes but let him do the finishing touch: Start the coat zipper but let him zip it up, or button all but one of his buttons.

Keep a stool handy so the child can see herself in the bathroom mirror. On the sink, keep a kid-sized hairbrush and toothbrush within arm's reach. Even if she resists brushing teeth and hair, be firm. Some things in life are nonnegotiable.

SNACK AND MEAL TIME

Provide a chair that allows the child's elbows to be at table height and feet to be flat on the floor. A stool or pillow may help. (Kids fidget less when they feel grounded.)

Offer a variety of ways to eat food, e.g., eat pudding with a spoon, or scoop it up with fingers; use a spoon or a fork to eat corn kernels, or use both hands to munch corn on the cob; and spoon chicken broth, or lift the bowl to her mouth.

Offer a variety of foods with different textures: lumpy, smooth, crunchy, chewy. Keep portions small, especially when introducing new foods.

Let the child pour juice or milk into a cup. A tipless cup will help prevent accidents. The child who frequently overreaches or spills juice needs much practice.

Encourage the child to handle snack-time or mealtime objects. Opening cracker packages, spreading peanut butter, and eating with utensils are good for proprioception, bilateral coordination, and fine-motor skills.

CHORES

Together, make a list of chores he can do to help around the house: Make his bed, walk the dog, empty wastebaskets, take out trash, pull weeds, rake, shovel, sweep, vacuum, fold laundry, empty the dishwasher, set and clear the table. Let him know you need and appreciate him. Make a routine and stick to it. If the child is forgetful, make a chart and post it on the refrigerator. When he finishes a chore, let him stick a star on the chart. Reward him with a special privilege or outing when he accumulates several stars. Break chores down into small steps. Let her clear the table one plate at a time. (She doesn't have to clear all the dishes.)

BATHING

Let the child help regulate the water temperature. Provide an assortment of bath toys, soaps, and scrubbers. Scrub the child with firm, downward strokes. Provide a large bath sheet for a tight wrap-up.

SLEEPING

Give your child notice: "Half an hour until bedtime!" or "You can draw for five more minutes."

Stick to a bedtime routine. Include stories and songs, a look at a sticker collection, a chat about today's events or tomorrow's plans, a back rub and snug tuck-in.

Children with tactile defensiveness are very particular about clothing, so provide comfortable pajamas. Some like them loose, some like them tight; some like them silky, some don't like them at all. Nobody likes them bumpy, scratchy, lacy, or with elasticized cuffs.

Use percale or silk sheets for a smooth and bumpless bed.

Let your child sleep with extra pillows and blankets, in a sleeping bag or bed tent, or on a waterbed.

Life at home can improve with a sensory diet and attention to your child's special needs, and life at school can improve as well.

Chapter Ten

YOUR CHILD AT SCHOOL

Becoming an advocate for your child, communicating with school personnel, finding a good school-and-child match, and sharing ideas with teachers can all promote your child's success at school.

WHAT A DIFFERENCE
COMMUNICATION MAKES!

Last year, Nicky hated fourth grade. Mrs. Colladay, his teacher, was mean. She always scolded him when he was slow, disorganized, or fidgety. She would say, "I wish you'd just try harder." He *was* trying.

This year, Nicky loves fifth grade. Ms. Berry is nice. She makes sure he understands the assignments and shows him how to break them down into manageable parts. She got him a chair that doesn't wiggle and thick pencils that don't break. She made him captain of the Flying Aces Math Team. She never makes him miss recess. She likes him.

* * *

What a difference a teacher makes! And what a difference a parent makes when she becomes her child's advocate!

Nicky is in a classroom that meets his needs because his mother took action. After years of seeking to avoid stigma and labels, she decided to inform the school about his sensory processing problems and about the benefits of therapy and a sensory diet. If Nicky could function more smoothly at home, surely he could gain confidence and competence at school.

During the summer, Nicky's mother met with the principal and Ms. Berry and was relieved to find them eager for information. They wanted to understand Nicky's strengths and weaknesses, so they could promote his success. They told her they would explain his needs to the art, science, and physical education teachers. They would arrange for special services at school. They would call her with questions and would welcome her calls.

What a difference communication makes!

If Only School Were
More Like Home

The child with SPD often has enormous difficulty in the classroom. His problem is not a lack of intelligence or willingness to learn. His problem may be dyspraxia, which is difficulty in knowing what to do and how to go about doing it.

The preschooler who has difficulty stringing beads often becomes the school-age child who can't organize the parts of a research project. He wants to interact successfully with the world around him, but he can't easily adapt his behavior to meet increasingly complex demands.

The out-of-sync child may be unable to settle down to work. Everything may be distracting—the proximity of a classmate, the sound of rustling paper, the movement of children playing outside the window, the scratchy label inside his shirt collar, and even the classroom furniture. He may be disorganized in his movements, verbal responses, and interactions with teachers and classmates.

For many reasons, school may be grueling:

1) School puts pressure on children to perform and conform. While the average child buckles down to meet expectations, the out-of-sync child buckles under pressure.

2) The school milieu is ever-changing. Abrupt transitions from circle time to art projects, from math to reading, or from cafeteria to gymnasium may overwhelm the child who switches gears slowly.

3) Sensory stimuli may be excessive. People mill around. Lights, sounds, and odors abound. The child may become overloaded easily.

4) Sensory stimuli may be insufficient. A long stretch of sitting may pose problems for the child who regularly needs short stretch breaks to organize his body. A spoken or written lesson, directed toward aural and visual learners, may not reach the kinesthetic and tactile learner.

5) School administrators and teachers often misunderstand SPD. They may be truly interested in helping the child, but they can't accommodate his unique learning style if they don't know where to begin.

6) School is not like home. For many children, school is unpredictable and risky, while home is familiar and safe.* The behavior of the child will differ because the environments differ. School can become more like home, however, when parents share information about their child with the adults who can make a difference in the child's success.

Years ago, before we became savvy about sensory processing, the St. Columba's director and I met with Allen's mother to learn

---

*(On the other hand, sometimes school is orderly and predictable, while home is stressful and chaotic.)

how we could help her boy. At preschool, he hardly spoke, hardly moved. He would park himself in the sandbox corner, behind a barricade of trucks. He had no self-help skills, no playmates, no affect. We described a sad, scared, helpless loner.

His mother was astonished. "But he isn't that way at all!" she said. Her description was 180 degrees different from ours. At home, he was a chatterbox. He was lively and cheerful. He jumped on the furniture, dug in the garden, and played with neighborhood kids. True, the kids he played with were all younger. True, he had trouble getting dressed. True, he had definite likes and dislikes in foods and activities. But he wasn't a problem at home. "If only school were more like home," she said with a sigh.

The conference was an eye-opener for everyone. As we talked, his mother realized that Allen functioned well at home because she fulfilled his need for consistent routines, just-right stimulation, physical security, and constant reminders of love. We, the teachers, realized that we could fulfill some of those needs at school, now that we understood what they were.

We entered a home-and-school partnership to help Allen succeed. The teachers became more sensitive to his cautious behavior and learned to guide him gently into preschool activities. They gave him more structure and protected him from overstimulation. Many small changes had a big, positive effect on his behavior.

Meanwhile, his mother adapted Allen's home environment to meet his special needs. She purchased some sensory-motor equipment, such as a trampoline, crawling tunnel, and Rainy Day Indoor Playground set (www.playawaytoy.com) and turned the basement into a mini-gym. She also became aware of her obligation to share her observations, selectively, with his school and teachers.

DECIDING WHOM TO TELL

The out-of-sync child needs an articulate advocate. Usually, it is up to a parent to make teachers and other caregivers aware of his special needs.

The thought of revealing their child's difficulties makes many parents anxious. They worry that the child may be stigmatized and labeled, that they may be blamed for the child's behavior, or that insensitive school personnel may be indiscreet or may use the information in the wrong way. Besides, talking about the child's inadequacies is painful. Nonetheless, for the child's sake, communication is essential.

Why is it necessary to provide information? Adults who work with children, like sculptors who work with clay, must have a feel for the material they shape. With some understanding of Sensory Processing Disorder, they can become more attuned to the child's differing abilities. Without information, however, they can't be expected to change their classroom environment, alter their teaching style, or redirect their thinking.

Who needs to know? Classroom teachers should be informed. The principal; the art, science, music, and physical education teachers; and the computer and media specialists may need to know. School bus and carpool drivers, religious school teachers, scout leaders, coaches, and baby-sitters also may be more considerate when told.

What information should be shared? Briefly, tell the teacher what the child's problem is. (Avoid terms such as "underresponsivity to vestibular sensations," unless pressed for details.) Then, give specific suggestions about what works at home, so the teacher can consider doing the same at school.

Examples: "My daughter is very sensitive to being touched or jostled. At home, we've noticed she does best when she doesn't feel crowded. Would you remember her need for space when you plan the seating arrangement?" Or, "My son has difficulty with motor coordination. He is receiving therapy to help him move more smoothly. At home, we find that frequent breaks to move and stretch help him get organized."

When you find that the teacher is receptive, you may also choose to share your own documented observations, therapists' evaluations, sensory diet suggestions, and tips for teachers, included at the end of this chapter.

How should information be shared? Frame the information positively: "She concentrates beautifully if . . . ," or "His motor coordination improves when. . . ." Stress the child's abilities: "She adores art projects," or "He has a great sense of humor." Enlist the teacher's goodwill: "We hope we can work together. Please keep me posted!"

Where should information be shared? Arrange meetings in advance, so you and the teacher can talk uninterrupted. Confer in the classroom before or after school, in the teachers' lounge at lunchtime, or by telephone at night.

When should information be shared? Before the school year starts, anticipate your child's difficulties and communicate with those who need to know. Help them be proactive, rather than reactive, when problems arise.

A GOOD SCHOOL-AND-CHILD MATCH

Communicating regularly with school personnel should make a positive difference for your child. Sometimes, however, the teacher will resist taking suggestions and making accommodations, even if your child is legally entitled to them. You will then have to decide whether to step in or step back.

For instance, one mother knew that chewing gum helped her son get organized while reading and writing. She asked the teacher if gum would be permissible. The teacher refused: "He can't have special privileges, just because he has special needs." Although the mother was reluctant to go over the teacher's head and make a fuss, she decided to complain to the principal. The principal intervened, the teacher relented, and the child was allowed to chew (but not crack) gum. His performance improved, and, several months later, the teacher apologized.

Sometimes, the teacher is willing to make adjustments, but the school resists. The child may benefit from a therapy ball seat instead of a chair, or a desk of his own rather than a shared table, or a locker he can open easily, while the school insists on regulation furnishings. In such cases, pick the most important battles—and keep fighting.

If goodness-of-fit at school is lacking, you have several options:

• Ask to move the child to another teacher's classroom.

• Investigate special-education programs. Special-education classes are smaller and less distracting than regular classrooms. Special educators are trained to address children's differing abilities. With an IEP (Individualized Education Program), the out-of-sync child may flourish.

• Transfer the child from one public school to another. An advantage of public education is the availability of facilities, including OTs, speech therapists, and remedial reading specialists. If the child is eligible for special education, these services are provided during the school day, at no charge.

• Enroll the child in a private school, with smaller class size and more individualized attention. In a private school the immature child can repeat a grade, if necessary, whereas in a public school the child may not get this chance to "pause" before promotion to a more challenging grade.

• Homeschool your child. Many children learn best at home, where they can go at their own pace without distractions. Participating in after-school activities is still your child's right and is also a good idea to encourage social interactions with other children.

Each school year, reopen the channels of communication. Teachers will come and go—some sensitive, some not so sensitive—and your steady support and voice will help your child succeed.

Below you will find some classroom strategies to share with your child's teacher. He or she may learn from these guidelines how to be supportive, how to gauge when to encourage and when to step back; how to refrain from overloading the child with excessive stimulation and unmanageable work; and how to control his or her own frustrations when dealing with an out-of-sync child.

Promoting Your Child's Success at School

The child with SPD needs understanding and support if he is going to succeed at school, whether that school is public or private. A teacher may want to help an out-of-sync student but may lack training in the appropriate techniques. If so, the teacher may wish to try some of the following classroom strategies that will help the out-of-sync child. They also help every other child.

Yes, every child!

Every child benefits from a safe, calm, and distraction-free environment. Every child requires frequent breaks from work to move and stretch. Every child needs to know that someone is paying attention to his strengths and weaknesses, likes and dislikes, ups and downs. Every child needs to be shown how to find solutions to problems. Every child needs assurance that it's okay to have differing abilities, that he can be successful, that his ideas have merit, that his personhood is valued.

When the out-of-sync child begins to feel more in control, his schoolwork and social skills will improve. When he is less distracted, he distracts the other children less. Then, when all the students are working to their best ability, the teacher can teach!

Classroom Strategies

CONTROLLING THE ENVIRONMENT

Reduce sensory overload. You may have to intuit what kind of sensory stimulation is getting in the child's way, because he may be unable to tell you. Remember that stimuli that bother him today may not bother him tomorrow, and vice versa. If you can remove or diminish most distractions, you will increase the child's ability to attend to the important job of learning. Help the child focus on one idea at a time by minimizing unrelated sensory stimuli. Simplify, simplify, simplify.

Tactile distractions may divert the child's attention. If the proximity of classmates irritates the child, help him find a spot where he will feel safe. Steer the younger child to a seat at the head of the table, or at the edge of the rug, to lessen the possibility of contact with other children. Station the older child's desk in a classroom corner, or up front near you.

Let her bring up the rear when the class tiptoes single file down the corridor so that no one can bump her from behind. Provide her with the space she needs.

Visual distractions may interfere with the child's concentration. Eliminate clutter on bulletin boards. Secure artwork, maps, and graphics on the walls so they don't flutter. Tack a sheet over open shelves to cover art materials, games, and toys that may attract the child's attention. Remove mobiles swaying from light fixtures. Adjust window blinds to prevent sunshine from flickering through.

The movements of other children may also be visually distracting. Have the child sit near you at the front of the room, with his back to his classmates. Surround him with children who sit quietly, pay attention, and serve as good role models.

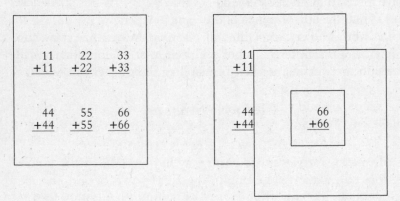

When preparing worksheets for the school-age child, keep to a minimum instructions to read and math problems to solve. White space around each written problem helps the child focus on one at a time. He may do best when he can frame each problem with a cardboard template.

Auditory distractions may make the room seem like an echo

chamber for the child with auditory processing problems. A classroom's hard surfaces, such as desktops, linoleum tiles, and painted walls, reflect sound. Wherever possible, cover hard surfaces with carpet, cloth, or corkboard. Be sure the child isn't seated near the humming fish tank, under the buzzing fluorescent bulb, or beside the window where he may be distracted by children's voices outside.

When the children are working at their desks, you may find that playing classical music, such as Bach and Mozart, softens the auditory environment and helps organize everybody.

Olfactory distractions may include the smells coming from the lunchroom or from the gerbil cage. If it is possible to adjust the schedule, time your lessons so that the child's most difficult subject is not being taught as the fragrance of grilled cheese wafts through the door. Keep animals, paint supplies, and other aromatic materials away from the child's desk.

Provide comfortable furniture. This prescription may be hard to fill for a teacher who must make do with regulation chairs and desks. However, the child who frequently falls off his chair because of inefficient body awareness may be able to align his body and maintain stable posture if the furniture fits.

Find the child a chair that does not tip, or stabilize it by jamming the legs into tennis balls. The height of the chair should allow him to place his feet flat on the floor. The height of the desk should be at his waist level.

An older child who is expected to sit at a desk for long periods might benefit from a textured cushion that will help him stick to the seat.* If the other students want to try the cushion, let them. Soon they'll forget about it, and you can get on with your job while the child who needs it stays put.

Sometimes, a special type of chair helps. If the preschooler is fidgety at circle time, for instance, a ball to sit on will help focus his attention. The ball's diameter should equal the distance be-

---

* A teenage boy, whose sensory problems had been overlooked for years, glued thumbtacks—points UP—to the seat of his desk chair at home. The tacks, he explained, reminded him when he was about to slide off the chair! A cushion would seem to be a preferable alternative.

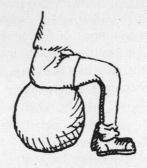

tween his buttocks and the floor when his knees are bent at a right angle and his feet are flat on the floor.

Keep chalkboards and worksheets clean. Fuzzy lines present problems for the child with visual processing difficulties. Most helpful are crisp white lines on a dark chalkboard and clear, dark lines on white paper so that the child can discriminate between the background and the letters or numbers you want her to understand.

MANAGING THE CLASSROOM

Develop a consistent routine. The out-of-sync child may have trouble getting organized to do what is necessary. He may struggle to overcome a feeling of chaos, internally and externally. Thus, he is most comfortable when things are "just so," exactly as they were yesterday and will be tomorrow. His rigidity is a manifestation of his need to organize his world.

For this child, a classroom that is clearly structured is preferable to one that runs on spontaneity. Help him by writing classroom routines on the board, sticking to the schedule, keeping the room arranged in a predictable way, and remembering whose turn it is to be line leader or to play with the new set of magnets.

Plan transitions as carefully as lessons. If focusing on a task is difficult, changing focus is even harder for the out-of-sync child.

Notify students about impending transitions: "In ten minutes, we'll go to the all-purpose room," or "After recess, you'll get the new reading books." Give plenty of notice when something out-of-the-ordinary will occur, such as a field trip, a visit from a reptile trainer, or a change in seating arrangements.

To facilitate transitions, signify what will happen next by clapping or beating drum rhythms. For instance, two long claps followed by three short claps may say that it is time to put away math books and stand up to stretch.

$$\overline{\quad} \quad \overline{\quad} \quad - \quad - \quad -$$

long,   long,   short,   short,   short

A sequence of one long clap followed by four short claps and a final long clap may mean that it is time to come in off the playground.

$$\overline{\quad} \quad - \quad - \quad - \quad - \quad \overline{\quad}$$

long,   short,   short,   short,   short,   long

Prepare transition fillers to turn empty time into teachable moments. Recite poems and sing activity songs with motions. Offer activities to strengthen language and critical-thinking skills, such as passing around laminated "What's Missing?" pages from children's magazines, or playing "What If?" games (What if we had wings? What if we had no electricity?).

Brainstorm together. Write down everyone's suggestions for class plays or for science projects. Assure each child that his idea is valid.

Take a vote. Who wants a happy face on the jack-o'-lantern, and who wants a scary face? Who hopes the Democrat will win, and who chooses the Republican? Who wants to study rain forests, and who prefers deserts?

Plan movement breaks between and during activities. Provide acceptable ways for the fidgety child to move. Incorporate movement into the routine, so children can stand and stretch, or move across the room from math to science center, or march to a drumbeat. Try activities such as "Simon Says" (where nobody loses), "Follow the Leader," "Jumping Jacks," or relay races. Play "Silent Speed Ball," in which the children pass a ball quickly around a circle, without making a peep. Movement helps every child pay attention, think, speak, and write.

Devise team or club efforts. Teams that read the most books, solve the most math problems, or produce cooperative projects earn a reward that you can decide on together. Earning team points can be a strong incentive for out-of-sync students, as well as for better organized classmates who may not choose to work with them.

HELPING CHILDREN BECOME
BETTER ORGANIZED

Encourage students to be active rather than passive learners. All children have an inner drive to learn, and they learn best when they can move and touch. Remember that reading and listening are not every child's main avenue of learning. Therefore, provide multisensory lessons so that the learning arrives through every possible route.

For example, the preschooler with inefficient auditory processing may learn best through tactile and visual experiences. Thus, he may learn more about rhythm and pitch by playing "Jingle Bells" on the xylophone than by hearing a recording. The older child, whose visual processing problem makes worksheets a chore, may learn well in hands-on, real-life situations. Thus, he can absorb math concepts while making change in a school store.

Many out-of-sync children have narrow interests. Find out what the child has an affinity for, and lead her to explore the subject she is passionate about, through her preferred sensory path. Is she interested in spiders? Planets? Native Americans? If she is a tactile learner, let her draw a picture or build a model. If she likes to talk, let her give a short oral presentation. If she loves to move, let her demonstrate ritual dances. Build on the child's sensory strengths. Then, give her books to read in the area in which she has expertise. Even prereaders learn best when they can investigate subjects that they consider interesting and relevant.

Post this Chinese proverb in your classroom as a constant reminder:

> *I hear, and I forget.*
> *I see, and I remember.*
> *I do, and I understand.*

Give children time. Nobody likes to feel rushed, especially the child with SPD who may take longer than others to process new information. This child needs warm-up time, just as much as cool-down time.

Give this child the luxury of time to learn new material:

A) Before presenting a lesson, tell the class what you will teach them,

B) Teach them,

C) Tell them what you have taught them, and then

D) Allow them time to absorb the lesson or to practice it. Drill is particularly valuable for the child who, lacking an internal sense of order, requires repetition of academic tasks before catching on.

Give the child time to process a question and answer. The special child often has the knowledge but just takes longer to prove it. Ten seconds is not too long to wait for an answer that someone else may produce in three.

Simplify instructions. When you give instructions, make eye contact with the child if possible. (Children with SPD or autism frequently are uncomfortable with eye contact and can listen better when they are not forced to look you in the eye.) Give one or two directions at a time. Be concise and specific. Repeat the instructions if necessary. When assigning daily homework, say it in words and put it in writing. Have the child repeat it and write it down herself.

Short assignments will match the child's short attention span, will help him see an end to the task, and will give him a series of little successes.

Break down big assignments into small chunks. He may be a great reader but have difficulty planning long-term research projects. Provide a schedule and your clear expectations. For example, Week 1: Each child will tell you his chosen topic. Week 2: He will submit a tentative reading list. Week 3: An outline. Week 4: A rough draft. Week 5: A finished report.

Provide a choice of writing implements. Some children do better with standard pencils, others with fat primary pencils; some with standard crayons, others with chubby crayons. While fine-motor skills generally develop later in boys than in girls, these skills are especially late-blooming in the boy or girl with SPD. Help the child choose the writing tool that fits him or her best.

Respect the child's needs. The child's primary need is to feel safe. When he feels safe, his brain is available for learning.

Many fine teachers, with the best intentions, commonly err with out-of-sync children by trying to jolly them out of their difficulties. For instance, a teacher may tell the preschooler with tactile overresponsivity that "everyone likes finger paint, so take your turn," hoping to change his tendency to withdraw from touch. A physical education teacher of the older child with vestibular overresponsivity may try to position him to do a somersault on the tumbling mat. These encouragements won't "fix" the child's dysfunction but, instead, may cause an aversive response, because he feels threatened.

Unless you know exactly what you're doing, it is better to respect the child's sensory defensiveness. Remember that the child's behavior is out of line not because he won't do things right but because he can't. It is unfair to force the child to do things he is unready to do.

Give the child alternatives. Anticipate problems, and help the child find suitable alternatives to situations that cause problems. For example, the child who is uncoordinated may avoid boisterous recess games. Guide him to other activities he can excel in that will strengthen his motor skills and that won't make him feel like a bystander or a sissy.

For the preschooler, going through an obstacle course at his own pace, after everyone else has completed it, is one possibility. If he resists a particular obstacle, such as the balance beam or tunnel, let him be! Praise him for conquering the obstacles he can manage.

For the older child, ball skills may improve after playing tetherball, one-on-one catching and throwing games, or dribbling activities with a teacher or a buddy.

In the classroom, the child who is easily distracted by too many choices may seem unable to choose any. He may say he's bored, when he is really confused. Help him find an activity or project that he can do while socializing with just one or two other children.

If possible, consult with an occupational therapist about classroom modifications, educationally relevant activities, and sensory-motor techniques you can use to address the child's needs during the school day.

ADAPTING YOUR OWN BEHAVIOR

Emphasize the positive. Give each child what psychotherapist Carl R. Rogers calls "unconditional, positive regard." The out-of-sync child needs constant assurance that her efforts are appreciated and worthwhile. She may not feel competent, even when she is! Reward the child for what she did accomplish, rather than remarking about what she left undone. Success breeds success.

Keep your voice low. The child with a supersensitive auditory system can become very uncomfortable when he hears a high-pitched or loud voice. He may even misinterpret your tone of voice and become distraught.

One day, I had to use a more forceful voice than usual to move a group of preschoolers through a Halloween song in which different rhythm instruments represent witches, skeletons, and pumpkins. Midway through the song, I raised my voice to be heard: "Now, please put down your tambourines and pick up your wood blocks."

I didn't understand then, although I do now, why a particularly anxious boy cried, "Don't talk to me that way! Don't you know I can't do anything right when you talk to me that way?" My words hadn't been threatening; my directions hadn't been complicated. It was my louder, higher voice that made him fall apart. More effective would have been whispering, the technique I use now, especially in a noisy room.

Provide physical feedback. When you want to be certain that the child is paying attention, get up close. Look the child in the eye, if possible. While speaking, put your hands on the child's shoulders and press down firmly. These techniques may help the child focus better on what you are saying.

Keep your expectations realistic. So what if the child doesn't complete a task or doesn't do it the way other children do? Remember what is most important in learning: process rather than product, and participation rather than perfection.

Chapter Eleven

COPING WITH YOUR
CHILD'S EMOTIONS

For the child to become more self-regulated and for families to deal with the emotional fallout of SPD, there are positive words and actions that may improve the child's skills and self-esteem, as well as pitfalls to avoid.

A TYPICALLY DREADFUL MORNING

Marge, the mother of two, tells this story:

> This morning was typically dreadful. Chip, my eight-year-old, got out of bed on the wrong side. Actually, he fell out of bed. Then, on his way to the bathroom, he crashed into Melissa and knocked her down. He yelled at her, "You're always in my way, dumb head!" She ran downstairs, bawling. He's always so mean to her, and she's only three.
>
> While I comforted her, I heard Chip slamming his bureau drawers and shouting. He finally came downstairs wearing his T-shirt inside out. He said this way the tags wouldn't

hurt him. I thought that was pretty good problem solving, but my husband disagreed. Before I could say anything, he ordered Chip to change. Chip refused. My husband was furious. He pulled off Chip's shirt, turned it right side out and stuffed Chip into it. Chip was really upset and fighting back tears.

Finally, he sat down and poured orange juice over his cereal. When I said that wasn't a good idea, he began to cry. He said, "It was an accident! I didn't do it on purpose!" Then he poured the rest of the juice on Melissa's head. On purpose.

Okay. I kept my temper, because it was time to meet the school bus. But Chip couldn't find his reading book. It took ten minutes to find it behind the couch. He missed the bus, so I drove him to school. When we got there, we saw a classmate getting out of her car. She had a model of an igloo made of sugar cubes. Then Chip really lost control. He had forgotten about the "Homes around the World" assignment. I felt just awful because I had forgotten, too. Chip hunkered down and refused to get out of the car.

The girl's mother waved to me and said, "These special projects take a lot out of me! What a dreadful morning!"

If she only knew!

What do we see here? Poor motor coordination. Tactile overresponsivity. Sibling rivalry. Conflict between parents. Anger. Rage. Frustration. Loss of autonomy. Poor self-help skills. Passive aggression. Disorganization. Loss of self-control. Defiance. Helplessness. Despair. Guilt. Inadequacy. Isolation.

If you have an out-of-sync child, these problems may be all too familiar. The effects of SPD can permeate your lives.

Is it possible to learn to cope with the emotional fallout? Yes, if you understand your child, if you have support and understanding, and if you educate yourself.

OTHER EXPERTS' ADVICE

Here are parenting techniques from Drs. Ayres, Greenspan, Silver, and Turecki, and from Mary Kurcinka and Maryann Colby Trott. Their ideas may help you develop consistent and positive coping skills. (See Selected Bibliography, p. 333.)

Pay Attention to Your Child

Remember that the child's problem is a physical one. Just as another child with measles can't help itching, the out-of-sync child can't help being clumsy or afraid.

Tune in to the kinds of stimulation that the child avoids or craves.

Find the best way to reach your child, through his preferred sensory channel. Use a variety of ways to communicate (talking, writing, drawing, gesturing, and demonstrating). Keep your messages simple.

Identify your child's temperament, by analyzing traits such as activity level, distractibility, intensity, regularity, sensory threshold, flexibility, and mood.

Know your child's strengths and weaknesses. If your child has been diagnosed, study the evaluations carefully. Read everything you can. Get information from teachers and specialists who are familiar with differing abilities and learning styles.

Set up Floortime, Stanley Greenspan's term for an unstructured, special play time, at least thirty minutes daily. Sit on the floor and let your child choose and lead the activity. Follow along in the play, paying attention to whatever interests him. Engaging with your child on his terms establishes a warm, trusting attachment, the basis of all future relationships. (See www.floortime.org.)

Anticipate Responses

Anticipate emotional crises. Too much stimulation at a birthday party or a crowded mall may trigger a negative response. Be ready to remove the child from sensations that will overwhelm her, before she loses control.

Help the child learn to notice her increasing intensity and need for space. Give her opportunities to remove herself from the action and to recharge by being alone.

Develop strategies with your child to cope with negative emotions before they occur. "Let's lay out your clothes tonight, so in the morning you won't feel rushed."

To diffuse her strong reactions, be prepared to provide soothing activities, such as a bath, story, quiet imaginative play, rocking chair, back rub, or trip to the playground.

If she is slow to react to sensory stimuli, allow her extra time before responding.

Empathize

Identify and empathize with the child's point of view, motives, and goals to help you understand his behavior, so you will have an easier time changing it.

Understand the child's feelings and reflect them back: "It's hard to sleep when you're worried about the monster in the closet." Reflective listening helps him identify and master his emotions.

Reassure him repeatedly that you understand his difficulties.

Share your own similar emotions, to show that we all have fears. "I think roller coasters are scary, too," or "We both get nervous in crowds."

Take time to reevaluate your child's emotions. He may be aggressive because he is afraid, not angry. Respond to the primary emotion, rather than to the defensive behavior.

Give your child coping skills for regaining self-control. After an emotional storm, provide a quiet space, firm hug, or walk, or appropriate words or actions to use to restore harmony. "Do you need to do something to feel better about what happened?"

Accentuate the positive. Comment about his abilities, interests, and good behavior. Build his self-concept by reinforcing his growing self-awareness and accomplishments.

Build on his strengths and help him compensate for his weaknesses. Welcome him to the world; do not excuse him from life.

Provide Structure

Establish consistent routines and schedules. Explain daily plans. Give notice of upcoming activities. Avoid surprises.

Limit transitions as much as possible. Allow time to end one activity before moving on to the next.

Expect the child to take longer than others to adapt to routines.

Help your child become organized in his own work. Together, set up schedules and job charts. Eliminate distractions. Provide sufficient space, time, and guidance to complete projects and homework, so he has the satisfaction of doing his work independently.

Have Realistic Expectations

Sometimes, your child may function well, and other times, she will resist going to school, spill her milk, and fall. Expect inconsistency. When she stumbles, try to be understanding.

Break challenges into small pieces. Encourage her to achieve one goal at a time to feel the satisfaction of a series of little successes.

Remember that you have had years of experience in learning to deal with the world, and that the child has not.

Discipline

When the child loses control, avoid punishment. Loss of self-control is scary enough; punishment adds guilt and shame.

Comment on the child's negative behavior, not on the child: "Your yelling makes me angry," rather than "You infuriate me!"

Help the child find a quiet space, away from sensory overload, as a technique to regain self-control. Let him decide the length of the time-out, if possible.

Set limits, to make a child feel secure. Pick one battle at a time to help him develop self-control and appropriate behavior.

Be firm about the limits you set. Show him that his feelings won't change the outcome; a rule is a rule. "I know you're mad because you want to play with the puppy, but it is suppertime."

Discipline consistently. Use gestures and empathy to explain why you are disciplining him. (Discipline means to teach or instruct, not punish.) After you tell him what you are going to do, then do it.

Determine appropriate consequences for misbehavior. A natural consequence is best, because it is reasonable, factual, and you don't impose it: "If you skip breakfast, you will be hungry." A logical consequence, in which the child is responsible for the outcome of his behavior, is second best: "If you throw food, you must mop it up." An applied consequence, in which the punishment doesn't exactly fit the crime, is useful when nothing else works: "If you spit on the baby, you may not play with your friends," or "If you hit me, you may not watch TV."

Reward appropriate behavior with approval.

Problem-Solve

Set up problem-solving time to discuss problems, negotiate differences, and arrive at solutions with your child. Elevating his problem-solving ability helps him anticipate challenges, take responsibility, cope with his feelings, become a logical and flexible thinker, and learn to compromise. "What else can you do when you're angry besides throwing toys? Can you say, 'I don't like that!' and jump up and down?"

Ask him for advice on how you can help him.

Help your child find appropriate outlets for emotions. Let her know when she can scream, where she can let loose, and what she can punch. Teach her that some negative expressions are acceptable and safe, while others are inappropriate.

When the child's intense emotions overwhelm you, first get control of your own feelings. You will show that strong emotions are a fact of life; everyone must learn to cope, and he, too, can learn to calm himself.

Have fun together. Life does not need to be serious all the time.

If necessary, seek extra support to help with the "ripple effect" of your hard-to-raise child. Professionals can help you improve family life and relations with relatives, peers, and others outside your nuclear family.

Join an SPD Parent Connections support group to share child-rearing concerns with others. (See www.SPDnetwork.org.)

Become Your Child's Advocate

Educate adults who need to know about your child's abilities. Because SPD is invisible, people may forget or disbelieve that a significant problem affects your child. Your job is to inform them, so they can help your child learn.

Monitor your child's classroom and group activities. If you see that a teacher or coach is insensitive, uncooperative, or too demanding, take action.

Intervene when the child can't handle a stressful situation alone. Reinforce the message that asking for help is a positive coping strategy, not an admission of failure.

DOS AND DON'TS FOR COPING

Here are my suggestions for dealing with the out-of-sync child on a daily basis.

Please Do . . .

Do build on the child's strengths: "You are such a good cook! Help me remember what we need for our meat loaf recipe. Then, you can mix it." Or, "You have energy to spare. Could you run over to Mrs. Johnson's house and get a magazine she has for me?" Think "ability," not "disability."

Do build on the child's interests: "Your collection of rocks is growing fast. Let's read some books about rocks. We can make a list of the different kinds you have found." Your interest and support will encourage the child to learn more and do more.

Do suggest small, manageable goals to strengthen your child's abilities: "How about if you walk with me just as far as the mailbox? You can drop the letter in. Then I'll carry you piggy-back, all the way home." Or, "You can take just one dish at a time to clear the table. We aren't in a hurry."

Do encourage self-help skills: To avoid "learned helplessness," sponsor your child's independence. "I know it's hard to tie your shoes, but each time you do it, it will get easier." Stress how capable she is, and how much faith you have in her, to build her self-esteem and autonomy. Show her you have expectations that she can help herself.

Do let your child engage in appropriate self-therapy: If your child craves spinning, let him spin on the tire swing as long as he wants. If he likes to jump on the bed, get him a trampoline, or put a mattress on the floor. If he likes to hang upside down, install a chinning bar in his bedroom doorway. If he insists on wearing boots every day, let him wear boots. If he frequently puts inedible objects into his mouth, give him chewing gum. If he can't sit still, give him opportunities to move and balance, such as sitting on a beach ball while he listens to music or a story. He will seek sensations that nourish his hungry brain, so help him find safe ways to do so.

Do offer new sensory experiences: "This lavender soap is lovely. Want to smell it?" Or, "Turnips crunch like apples but taste different. Want a bite?"

Do touch your child, in ways that the child can tolerate and enjoy: "I'll rub your back with this sponge. Hard or gently?" Or, "Do you know what three hand squeezes mean, like this? I-Love-You!"

Do encourage movement: "Let's swing our arms to the beat of this music. I always feel better when I stretch, don't you?" Movement always improves sensory processing.

Do encourage the child to try a new movement experience: "If you're interested in that swing, I'll help you get on." Children with dyspraxia may enjoy new movement experiences but need help figuring out how to initiate them.

Do offer your physical and emotional support: "I'm interested in that swing. Want to try it with me? You can sit on my lap, and we'll swing together." The child who is fearful of movement may agree to swing at the playground if he has the security of a loving lap. (Stop if he resists.)

Do allow your child to experience unhappiness, frustration, or anger: "Wow, it really hurts when you don't get picked for the team." Acknowledging his feelings allows him to deal with them, whereas rushing in to make it better every time he's hurt prevents him from learning to cope with negative emotions.

Do provide appropriate outlets for negative emotions: Make it possible to vent pent-up feelings. Give her a ball or a bucketful of wet sponges to hurl against the fence. Designate a "screaming space" (her room, the basement, or garage) where she can go to pound her chest and shout.

Do reinforce what is good about your child's feelings and actions, even when something goes wrong: "You didn't mean for the egg to miss the bowl. Cracking eggs takes practice. I'm glad you want to learn. Try again." Help her assess her experience positively by talking over what she did right and what she may do better the next time. How wonderful to hear that an adult is sympathetic, rather than judgmental!

Do praise: "I noticed that you fed and walked the dog. Thanks for being so responsible." Reward the child for goodness, empathy, and being mindful of the needs of others. "You are a wonderful friend," or "You make animals feel safe."

Do give the child a sense of control: "If you choose bed now, we'll have time for a long story. If you choose to play longer, we won't have time for a story. You decide." Or, "I'm ready to go to the shoe store whenever you are. Tell me when you're ready to leave." Impress on the child that others don't have to make every decision that affects him.

Do set reasonable limits: To become civilized, every child needs limits. "It's okay to be angry but not okay to hurt someone. We do not pinch."

Do recall how you behaved as a child: Maybe your child is just like you once were. (The apple doesn't fall far from the tree!) Ask yourself what you would have liked to make your childhood easier and more pleasurable. More trips to the playground, free time, or cuddling? Fewer demands? Lower expectations? Try saying, "When I was a kid and life got rough, I liked to climb trees. How about you?"

Do respect your child's needs, even if they seem unusual: "You sure do like a tight tuck-in! There, now you're as snug as a bug in a rug." Or, "I'll stand in front of you while we're on the escalator. I won't let you fall."

Do respect your child's fears, even if they seem senseless: "I see that your ball bounced near those big kids. I'll go with you. Let's hold hands." Your reassurances will help her trust others.

Do say "I love you": Assure your child that you accept and value who she is. You cannot say "I love you" too often!

Do follow your instincts: Your instincts will tell you that everyone needs to touch and be touchable, to move and be movable. If your child's responses seem atypical, ask questions, get information, and follow up with appropriate action.

Do listen when others express concerns: When teachers or caregivers suggest that your child's behavior is unusual, you may react with denial or anger. But remember that they see your child away from home, among many other children. Their perspective is worth considering.

Do educate yourself about typical child development: Read. Take parent education classes. Learn about invariable stages of human development, as well as variable temperaments and learning styles. It's comforting to know that a wide variety of behaviors falls within the normal range. Then, you'll find it easier to differentiate between typical and atypical behavior. Sometimes a cigar is just a cigar, and a six-year-old is just a six-year-old!

Do seek professional help: SPD is a problem that a child can't overcome alone. Parents and teachers can't "cure" a child, just as a child can't cure himself. Early intervention is crucial.

Do keep your cool: When your child drives you crazy, collect your thoughts before responding, especially if you are angry, upset, or unpleasantly surprised. A child who is out of control needs the calm reassurance of someone who is in control. She needs a grown-up.

Do take care of yourself: When you're having a hard day, take a break! Hire a baby-sitter and go for a walk, read a book, take a bath, dine out, make love. Nobody can be expected to give another person undivided attention, and still cope.

Please Don't . . .

Don't try to persuade your child that he will outgrow his difficulties: "One day you'll climb Mt. Everest!" Growing older does not always mean growing stronger, or more agile, or more sociable. For children with SPD, growing older often means inventing new ways to avoid everyday experiences.

Don't tell your child she is bound to get stronger, better organized, or more in control, if she applies herself: "You can do better if you'll just try!" The child *is* trying.

Don't joke: "Why are you so tired? Did you just run a four-minute mile, ha ha?" Being tired is not a laughing matter to the child. Jokes make him feel laughed at and produce self-defeating anger and humiliation.

Don't plead: "Do it for Mommy. If you loved me, you'd sit up like a nice young lady." Your child does love you and yearns to please you, but she can't. Besides, she would sit up straight if she could, for her own sake, even if she didn't love you!

Don't shame: "A big boy like you can open the door all by himself." He may be big yet have little strength.

Don't threaten: "If you don't pick your feet up when you walk, then you'll ruin your shoes and you won't get any new ones." If/then threats backfire.

Don't talk about your child in demeaning ways in front of him: "This dopey-looking kid is my son. Wake up, Lazybones, and give our new neighbor a high-five!" Such comments aren't funny to the listener.

Don't talk about your child in demeaning ways behind his back: "My kid is such a lazy good-for-nothing. I just can't get him to understand the importance of hard work." What do you want your boss, relatives, and friends to remember about your child?

Don't compare, aloud, one child with another: "Your brother rode a two-wheeler when he was six. What's wrong with you?" (But do note to yourself the abilities your child seems to lack, compared with others of the same age.)

Don't do for your child what your child can do for himself: "I'll sharpen your pencils, while you get out your homework." Pampering a child gets you both nowhere fast.

Don't expect consistency: "You could hang your coat up yesterday. Why can't you do it today?" Inconsistency is common in out-of-sync children. What worked yesterday may not work today, and vice versa!

Don't make your child do things that distress him: "You must put your hand into this paint to make a handprint for Grandpa," or "You'll love riding the elevator up the Empire State Building." You can't make him enjoy touch or movement experiences until his neurological system is ready.

Don't overload your child with multisensory experiences: "Let's eat some chili, put on some steel-band music, and dance the rumba. We're going to have a terrific south-of-the-border night." Slow down! Offering your child a variety of sensations, one at a time, is fine; offering her a variety of sensations, all at the same time, will overload her system.

Don't be afraid of "labeling" your child: Many parents fear the stigma attached to SPD. They don't want their son or daughter to be labeled as a child with special needs. That fear is normal, but it doesn't help your child. Consider the identification of SPD as a benefit, for now you know that your child can get help before the problem turns into a serious learning disability.

Don't feel helpless: The world is full of children with SPD, and people who love them. You and your child are not alone. Support is out there; it awaits you, and you can find it.

Chapter Twelve

LOOKING AT YOUR CHILD
IN A NEW LIGHT

A PARENT'S EPIPHANY

A father writes, "When I first heard the words 'sensory integration' and 'low muscle tone' used in connection with my daughter Julie, I both didn't know what they meant and also dismissed them as yet another example of my wife's overprotectiveness. These terms were used by Stanley Greenspan, MD—one of the city's (and country's) top child psychiatrists—whom we had consulted on Julie's sleep problems. Such technical jargon was testimony, in my mind, to the unspoken alliance that surely persisted between high-paid child experts and jittery mothers.

"True, at twelve months, Julie did flop around a little more than I would have expected (she did not yet crawl or stand), and true, she didn't snuggle as I had hoped. But I chalked it up to her being a little prickly and thought she was fine just as she was. The fact is, I hadn't seen enough other kids (as my wife and the doctor had) to know that her behavior was out of the ordinary.

"While I was either objecting or standing aside, my wife persisted. She took Julie to an occupational therapist—also well paid and ready to agree with the diagnosis—and put Julie into a twice-a-week course of therapy. I remained skeptical.

"The turning point came when I attended a workshop called 'Understanding Sensory Integration.' While the presentation initially had limited impact on me, I was impressed with the number of parents there. 'So maybe this sensory stuff is for real,' I thought, 'and we're not the only ones who are concerned.'

"More important than the large turnout were the 'experience' stations in the back of the room. When I tried to accomplish simple tasks with some of my senses impaired—walking a straight line while looking through the wrong end of a pair of binoculars, for example—it started to penetrate my thick skull that Julie may in fact have entered the world with some special needs, and would have to compete with her peers at an unfair disadvantage as long as she had them.

"Suddenly, the significance of all this dawned on me—and I began to look at my daughter in a new light.

"From that point on, I became increasingly supportive of whatever would expand Julie's sensory and gross-motor horizons. I remember our glee when Julie started mashing food with her hands. I am now aghast that, out of ignorance and bravado, I would probably have denied Julie help at a critical time in her life, when she had her best chance to keep sensory deficiencies from becoming deep and lasting scars. And I applaud my wife who was forced to do battle on two fronts—Julie's deficiencies and my resistance—to allow Julie to overcome her deficiencies before she ever knew she had them."

BECOMING ENLIGHTENED

When you begin to understand Sensory Processing Disorder, you, too, will begin to look at your child in a new light. Recognizing that he is struggling to master the simplest tasks of everyday life is the first step toward helping him while he is still young.

Accepting your child's limitations isn't easy. It's natural to want to deny that your child's difficulties are out of the ordinary. It's natural to feel sad when you understand how hard he must work. It's natural to feel guilty for the times you scolded him or got impatient because of his behavior.

It takes time to become enlightened. It will take psychic and physical energy to begin the journey toward making him feel better about himself and about what he can achieve. If you're reading this, you are already on the road, so take heart. It's going to get better.

Your child is unable, not unwilling, to perform routine tasks. Maybe she often says that she is "just too tired." Maybe she slumps over the dining room table instead of sitting upright, or hasn't the energy to turn a doorknob, although she seems to be eating and sleeping enough.

Redirect your thinking: When she says she's tired, she means it. She really is unable—not unwilling—to perform routine tasks. No matter how much she wants to be independent and peppy, her sensory processing problem hinders her motoric ability. She knows, subconsciously, that her strength is limited. She has deduced how to reserve it for the jobs she knows she must do, which may be chewing, getting in and out of the car, or bending down to retrieve a dropped mitten.

Your child isn't lazy; in fact, she is using enormous energy just to get through the day.

Your child has developed some clever compensatory skills. Away from home, it could be that your child doesn't appear to be as smart as you know he is. He may not talk much, giving the impression that he has little to discuss. Conversely, he may talk non-stop, yet be a poor conversationalist.

He may seem uncommonly shy with unfamiliar adults and other children. He may choose the same old games and toys, as if he lacks curiosity and a sense of intellectual adventure.

Redirect your thinking: SPD affects all kinds of children, including those who are extremely intelligent. Give your child credit for being so bright that he has figured out how to avoid making a fool of himself when he knows he can't meet others' expectations.

Perhaps your child has lofty thoughts but can't express them well because of a language disability that is sometimes associated with vestibular dysfunction. Or, he may be verbally adept with a repertoire of excuses for evading intolerable movement or tactile experiences: "I can't paint today, because I'm wearing my new shirt and I shouldn't get it dirty."

Perhaps he has learned that if you see him digging in the sandbox, you will leave him alone. If he's busy, maybe you won't urge him to get on the swing, an activity that makes him feel that he is falling off the earth. You may notice that he looks up at you frequently, checking in for your approval, rather than concentrating on digging all the way to China.

Perhaps, if he can't climb stairs easily, he has figured out a way to get you to carry him. When a child reaches up two small arms for an embrace and says, "Hug me up the stairs," what parent would believe that neurological dysfunction is a problem?

Your child has developed compensatory skills that allow him to devise acceptable methods of avoiding the areas he knows will give him trouble.

Your child has courage. Perhaps your child resists descending the playground slide, doesn't like to play at other children's houses, shuns new foods, or becomes very anxious before visiting the doctor for an annual checkup. You may be exasperated by what you see as her excessive and inappropriate fearfulness.

Redirect your thinking: People need fear; fear alerts us to danger. Your child's apprehensions may seem excessive, but they are appropriate for her, because her world seems dangerous. Each day she must face the same scary situations, such as a fear of losing her balance or of being touched. No wonder she is cautious about new situations, which are even scarier because they are unpredictable.

Furthermore, it takes courage to resist enjoyable experiences, resist change, or resist a parent. The penalty for disappointing an important grown-up is disapproval. No one seeks disapproval. But disapproval is preferable to proceeding with an activity that the child perceives as life threatening.

Your child is brave, not a coward.

Your child has a tender heart. Perhaps your child has a "bad boy" reputation. He behaves aggressively, confronting the world with a stick in his hand, slugging the playmate who brushes against him, and shouting "I hate that!" "This is boring!" "You're stupid!" "Get away or I'll kill you!" These antagonistic responses may make your child appear to be a truly unpleasant person, even if you know that within the bully beats a tender heart.

Redirect your thinking: Perhaps your child can't differentiate between benign and hostile tactile experiences. Because he must protect himself from situations that he senses are dangerous, he instinctively chooses "fight" over "flight." He puts up a "don't mess with me" façade, not because he is misanthropic, but because he is scared.

The child who is inwardly on the defensive will often be outwardly offensive. An air of arrogance or a tough-guy image is common among people (adults, too) who feel uncertain about their abilities and self-worth.

You know how loving your child can be at home, in his familiar surroundings. He would be gentle outside the family circle, too, if he felt more comfortable in the world.

Your child has many abilities. Your child may not be skillful at reading, running, or paying attention. Her shortcomings may disappoint you.

Redirect your thinking: She may show extraordinary empathy and compassion for other living things. She may have a rare talent for creative thinking and be artistic, musical, or poetic. She may be observant where others are oblivious. She may have a wonderful sense of humor. Her special sensitivities may be a tremendous asset. Think abilities, not disabilities.

Your child has a special need for love and approval. Maybe she strikes you as being too possessive. She grabs all the toys but may not play with them; she just wants to have them. She demands all your time, but when you give it to her, she is unsatisfied. If she loses a round of Candyland, she cries and mopes. She wants it all.

Redirect your thinking: She requires things and attention to bolster her own small store of self-esteem. She has to be the winner because she usually feels like a loser. She seems greedy because she is needy.

More than anything, your child has a special need to be loved and appreciated.

Your child's "hardheadedness" is a survival skill. Perhaps he says things like "I'm the boss of my own body. You can't tell me what to do." Perhaps he is rigid, always wanting to wear the same clothes and eat the same cereal in the same bowl. Perhaps he insists on elaborate rituals for bath- or bedtime.

Redirect your thinking: Nobody awakens in the morning thinking, "Today I'm going to resist everything." Human beings learn to cope with a changing environment by being flexible. Your little fellow appears stubborn, however, because he is not the boss of his own body, and he is not in control. His life is full of uncertainties and obstacles.

An inefficient tactile system, with an attendant fussiness about clothing, may be the reason that he wants to wear shorts when it snows. Because the inside of his mouth may be overly sensitive to food textures, he may insist on the same kind of cereal, day after day.

Sameness and rituals are tools that help him accomplish basic jobs, like getting dressed or preparing for bed. His apparent stubbornness is rooted in his need to survive.

He isn't willfully stubborn; he is stubborn because he has trouble adapting his behavior to meet changing demands, so he sticks to what he knows will work.

Your child truly requires your attention, tailored to his needs. Let's suppose you dress your little boy in the morning, because he takes so long and becomes tearfully frustrated when you leave the job up to him. Then let's suppose that his preschool teacher mentions how much extra time is required for her to attend to his needs. She suggests that you urge him to become independent in the getting-dressed department. Even if you know more than she does about problems caused by SPD, you may still believe that your parenting skills are inadequate.

Redirect your thinking: Giving your child attention when he

needs it and when a job must get done quickly is perfectly okay. Particularly when your family runs on a tight schedule, you will do whatever works to move everybody from Point A to Point B.

Unenlightened parents ignore their children. Enlightened parents do what they can to make their children's lives pleasant and safe.

Your child can function better—with help. If your child has sensory difficulties now, her problems will grow with her. Certainly, she may develop strategies to avoid or compensate for stressful sensory experiences. Certainly, she may develop talents that are not dependent upon her shaky sense of balance, or hypersensitivity to touch. But she will always have to work very, very hard to function smoothly.

Redirect your thinking: SPD is like indigestion of the brain. Just as antacid can soothe upset stomachs, so can occupational therapy and a sensory diet smooth neural pathways.

Most of all, your everyday love and empathy will boost your child's emotional security. We all need to know that someone is there for us, especially when times are rough. We all need to know that someone applauds our strengths, understands our weaknesses, and honors our individuality. With your help, your son or daughter can become in sync with the world.

A PARENT'S ENCOURAGING WORDS

A mother writes: "If we had only known. If only there had been a book like this to read. If only our long- and eagerly awaited child had been 'normal.'

"Initially, we thought he was. He had great Apgar scores [measuring a newborn's condition] and was on schedule with all developmental checklists. Certainly, he had no obvious physical abnormalities; he was beautiful. Moreover, he was alert, learning to talk at six months! When he was two years old, all the pediatricians at the clinic dropped what they were doing to observe his phenomenal verbal skills. We were so proud.

"But at the same time, we knew that something was not right. Something had not been right all along. In the newborn nursery, he cried so loudly that he kept all the other babies awake. Then there was the traumatic transition from breast to bottle feeding. In fact, any kind of transition from one experience to another was horrendous.

"He was also extremely sensitive to light touch and new textures. It was difficult to dress him. Then came Gymboree, with terror and screaming at physical activities the other children loved. I had to face the stares from critical instructors and parents of more 'cooperative' children. With time, his behavior became more and more troublesome.

"What was wrong with my child? My beautiful and funny child.

"Finally, I contacted the public school's early childhood screening program, and we were scheduled for a group screening.

"When we arrived at the appointed time and place, we found many children with obvious handicaps and a play table to occupy them until their turn to go through the stations. Those with mental retardation, braces, and missing limbs went ahead smoothly.

"At our turn, the transition from play to screening activity resulted in a screaming, limp child who could not be handled by all the experts assembled. We left in tears. Our son, the only child with no discernible problem, couldn't even be tested.

"Upon subsequent individual evaluation by a team including an educational specialist, occupational therapist, speech pathologist, and psychologist, we were finally introduced to the 'something wrong.' Its name was Sensory Integration Dysfunction [Sensory Processing Disorder]. It required 'occupational therapy' and 'a good nursery school.'

"Why had it taken so long? Why hadn't *anyone* known? Why had my family suffered so much?

"It didn't matter now. The good nursery school was at hand.

"Upon the recommendation of the evaluation team, I contacted St. Columba's. I will never forget my first conversation with Carol Kranowitz. It was the first day my fear began to abate. She was the Music and Movement teacher, but she was so much more. She was the first person to whom I had ever spoken who knew my child without ever having met him. That is because she knew about SPD and had undertaken to inform and train other staff in its idiosyncrasies and, even more important, its management.

"These people at St. Columba's were not afraid of my child. They didn't see him as 'bad' or 'uncontrolled.' They saw him struggling with sensory processing problems, and though he challenged them mightily, they never gave up.

"With occupational therapy, we began to overcome such hurdles as fear of movement and revulsion caused by unfamiliar textures. As his fear of new things diminished, as the world became a less scary place, transitions also improved. With a psychologist's help, we structured the environment and managed behavioral responses (i.e., tantrums) consistently.

"Gradually, our child has blossomed and we have learned to do something with him which I never thought would be possible. We learned to enjoy him. He is our favorite companion.

"As I look back upon two years of OT and a nurturing nursery school, I shudder to think what a mess we would all have been without them. They were our lifeline, our hold on hope.

"Here is my charge to you: If you have concerns about your own or another child, no matter how vague they seem or how inarticulate you feel verbalizing them, pursue them. A child can have less pronounced problems than mine and still need help. And in your pursuit, continue until you find hope. In doing so, you may free other wonderful, enjoyable, little people held hostage by sensory processing problems. They are too small and frightened to free themselves."

APPENDIX A: THE SENSORY PROCESSING MACHINE

Here is a brief anatomy lesson about the central nervous system, and an explanation of how sensory processing occurs therein. This overview may help you appreciate the marvel of the brain-and-body connection.

THE SYNCHRONIZED NERVOUS SYSTEM

All animals respond to sensations of touch, movement and gravity, and body position. Thus, human animals share the hidden senses with goldfish and goats, falcons and frogs, caterpillars and clams. Through eons of evolution, humankind refined these senses in order to survive in a hazardous world.

As life forms gradually arose from sea to land to treetops, they had to adapt to differing environments. Hands to pluck berries, limbs to climb trees, eyes to see moving as well as stationary objects, and ears to detect prey and predators developed over time.

Along with these skills came increasingly complex sensations. The human brain evolved to process these sensations, so that the hand would pick a berry rather than a thorn, the limb would cling to a branch, the eye would discern a motionless tiger poised to pounce, and the ear would hear faraway hoof beats.

With the most complex brain in the animal kingdom, humans have the most complex nervous system. Its main task is to process sensations.

The nervous system has three main parts, working in harmony. One is the peripheral nervous system, running through organs and muscles, such as the eyes, ears, and limbs. The second part is the autonomic nervous system, controlling involuntary functions of heart rate, breathing, digestion, and reproduction. The third part is the central nervous system (CNS), consisting of countless neurons, a spinal cord, and a brain.

THREE COMPONENTS OF THE
CENTRAL NERVOUS SYSTEM

A) The Neurons

Neurons, or nerve cells, are the structural and functional units of the nervous system. Neurons tell us what is happening inside and outside our bodies. The brain has approximately 100 billion neurons. Each neuron has:

• A cell body, with its nucleus inside.

• Many short dendrites (Greek for "little branches") reaching out to other neurons to receive messages, or impulses, and carrying them into the cell body.

• A long axon, like a stem with roots, which sends impulses from the cell body to the dendrites of other neurons.

A Neuron

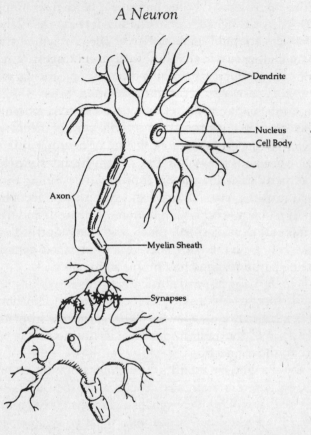

Two kinds of neurons connect the brain and spinal cord to the rest of the body: sensory and motor. Sensory neurons receive impulses from sensory receptors in our eyes, ears, skin, muscles, joints, and organs.

Impulses travel along the sensory neuron's axon and communicate messages to other neurons at contact points called synapses (Greek for "point of juncture"). Each neuron makes thousands of synaptic connections every time it fires. The neuron firing off the message is called presynaptic; the neuron receiving the message is called postsynaptic.

At the nanosecond that the message is fired, neurotransmitters are released, causing an electrochemical response. When neurotransmitters activate the receptors of the postsynaptic neurons, they are called excitatory. When they do not activate receptors, they are called inhibitory. (The process of balancing excitatory and inhibitory messages is called modulation. See p. 57)

The postsynaptic neurons may be other sensory neurons, or they may be motor neurons, the second kind of neurons in our CNS. Receiving the information, the motor neurons instruct muscles to move, glands to sweat, lungs to breathe, intestines to digest, and other body parts to respond appropriately.

In the growing fetus, neurons and synaptic connections multiply rapidly. A baby is born with billions of neurons and trillions of synapses. Sensations of smell, touch, and hunger activate synaptic connections to help the baby survive. For instance, synaptic connections help him respond to a nipple so he can suck.

To help the baby respond efficiently to this early skill of sucking, as well as to more complex skills, a process called myelination occurs. Myelin is a substance—somewhat like an electrical insulator—that coats the axon of the neuron to protect it, to smooth the path, and to speed up the connections.

At about eighteen months, the child stops developing new neurons, because his brain already has all that it needs—and his skull has all that will fit! New synapses, however, keep multiplying as the child integrates new sensations. That is, synapses multiply if synaptic connections are useful for everyday functioning and if they are repeatedly used. Otherwise, they vanish.*

By about twelve years, the child will lose many synapses he was born with, through a normal and necessary process called pruning. Pruning eliminates synapses the child does not need and stabilizes those he does. If he is Japanese, his brain will prune synapses necessary to pronounce the sound of "r," because "r"

---

* If a person doesn't engage in a wide range of sensory experiences, it becomes more difficult to use certain synaptic connections. For instance, when astronauts return to Earth after a few days, they have trouble reestablishing their sense of balance, because their gravity receptors were not stimulated in space.

isn't used in his language. If he is French, his brain will strengthen these synapses, so he can roll an "r" with fluency.

Normally, as the child actively responds to sensations, useful synaptic connections increase. The more connections, the more myelination; the more myelination, the stronger the neurological structure; and the stronger the neurological structure, the better equipped the child is to learn new skills.

TWO EXAMPLES OF THE FUNCTION OF NEUROTRANSMITTERS

City Sensations Become Routine

You leave your quiet country home and visit the city for the first time. The sound of traffic, the sight of crowds, the smell of pollution, and the motion of escalators bombard your senses. Billions of neurons are firing messages; zillions of neurotransmitters are activating neuronal responses. Your nervous system is operating on overtime; that's why you're so "nervous"!

After a few days, you begin to grow accustomed to city sensations. You no longer jump each time you hear screeching brakes or get jostled on the subway. Neurotransmitters now have less of an excitatory effect and more of an inhibitory effect. As your nervous system adapts to repeated stimuli, you can pay less attention to every sensation—and still survive.

Painkillers Become Less Effective

You have chronic back pain, so you take a painkiller. At first, the medicine helps as the neurotransmitters activate a response. After a while, the medicinal effect wears off because postsynaptic neurons have raised their threshold. Instead of just one painkiller to make you comfortable, you now require two or three.

B) The Spinal Cord

Extending below the brain is the spinal cord, a long, thick structure of nervous tissue. It receives all sensations from peripheral nerves in our skin and muscles and relays these messages up to the brain. The brain then interprets the sensory messages and sends motor messages back down to the spinal cord, which sends messages out to peripheral nerves in specific body parts.

C) The Brain

The human brain evolved over the course of 500 million years. Dr. Paul D. MacLean, brain researcher at the National Institute of Mental Health, has proposed that each human is born with a "triune brain." (This model of brain development is one of many. For our purposes, it is the simplest.)

As we evolved, we added layers of brain material, each one improving earlier parts. The first layer is the reptilian complex: the "primitive brain." It is responsible for reflexive, instinctive functions necessary for self-preservation and sexual drive. Sometimes these functions are called the "Four Fs": Feeding, Fighting, Fleeing . . . and sexual reproduction.

The Triune Brain

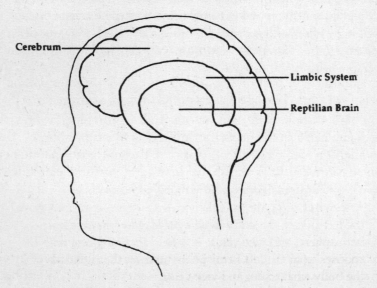

The second layer is the limbic system (Latin for "border"). It is the "seat of emotions," controlling hormones that enable us to feel angry, lustful, and jealous, as well as pleased and happy. Sometimes called the "smell brain," this system processes smell and taste, which have a powerful effect on our emotions.

The limbic system adds feelings to otherwise instinctive behavior. Thus, when we feel threatened, we fight or flee—or shut down. When we feel safe, we can play—and when we play, we can learn.

The third layer is the cerebrum: the "thinking brain." It is responsible for the organization of the most complex sensory intake. Detailed processing of sensations occurs here, so we can think, remember, make decisions, solve problems, plan and execute our actions, and communicate through language.

FOUR BRAIN PARTS USED
IN SENSORY PROCESSING

Four important brain structures are involved in sensory processing. Let's glance at them and see how they fit into the triune brain.

1. The Brain Stem

The brain stem, part of the "primitive brain," is an extension of the spinal cord. The brain stem performs four key functions.

- **A crossroads**, it receives sensory messages, particularly from skin and muscles in the head and neck, and relays this information to the cerebrum. In turn, the cerebrum sends out messages for motor coordination.

- **A switching gate**, it is the location where sensations from the left side of the body cross over to the right cerebral hemisphere, and vice versa. It is here that outgoing responses from the left hemisphere instruct the right side of the body what to do, and vice versa.

A Cross-Section of the Brain

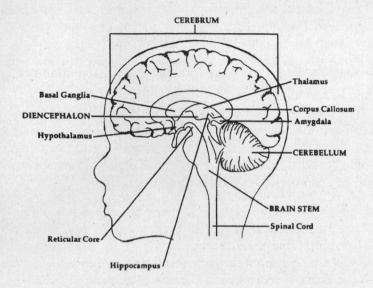

- **A clearinghouse**, it processes vestibular sensations necessary for hearing, maintaining our balance, seeing moving objects, and focusing our attention on one thing or another.

- **A regulator**, it processes sensations from internal organs and controls breathing, heartbeat, and digestion. It is the seat of the reticular core, a neuronal network that exchanges data with the vestibular system to guide our sense of timing for waking up, falling asleep, getting excited, and calming down.

2. The Cerebellum

Another part of the primitive brain is the cerebellum (Latin for "little brain"). Processing proprioceptive and vestibular sensations, it coordinates muscle tone, balance, and all our body movements. It controls fine-motor skills, especially repetitive movements, such as touch-typing and practicing scales. It lets us move easily, precisely, and with good timing. An Olympic diver has a finely tuned cerebellum that allows him to execute a seemingly effortless dive.

3. The Diencephalon

The diencephalon (Greek for "divided brain"), sometimes called the "tweenbrain," nestles in the center of the brain. A part of the limbic system, the diencephalon is associated with several important structures.

The basal ganglia are clusters of nerves that coordinate vestibular sensations necessary for balance and voluntary movement. The basal ganglia relay messages among the inner ear, the cerebellum, and the cerebrum.

The hippocampus (Greek for "sea horse," which it resembles) compares old and new stimuli. If it remembers a sensation, like the feel of comfortable shoes, it sends out inhibitory neurons to tell the cortex not to get aroused. If the sensation is new, like too-tight boots, it alerts the cortex with excitatory neurons.

The amygdala (Greek for "almond") connects impulses from the olfactory system and the cortex. It processes emotional memories, such as the smell of an old boyfriend's cologne, and influences emotional behavior, especially anger.

The hypothalamus controls the autonomic nervous system, regulating temperature, water metabolism, reproduction, hunger and thirst, and our state of alertness. It also has centers for emotions: anger, fear, pain, and pleasure.

The thalamus is the key relay station for processing all sensory data except smell. Thalamus means "couch" in Greek; it is where the cerebral hemispheres sit. Most sensations pass through it en route to our great gift, the cerebrum.

4. The Cerebrum

The most recently developed layer of the triune brain is the cerebrum (Latin for "brain"). Its wrinkled surface is the cerebral cortex (Latin for "bark"), often referred to as the neocortex because it is new, in evolutionary terms. The cerebrum is composed of two cerebral hemispheres.

Why do we need two hemispheres? One theory is that the right and left hemispheres developed when early humanoids lived in trees and learned to use one hand independently from the other. This was a useful survival skill: One hand could gather fruit while the other clung to a branch. Asymmetric use of the hands and asymmetric hemispheres in the brain developed together in a process called lateralization (from Latin for "side").

With lateralization came specialization. Specialization describes the different jobs of the two hemispheres. With discrete duties, the right and left hemispheres must work together for us to function at a high level.

In general, the left hemisphere is the cognitive side. It directs analytical, logical, and verbal tasks, such as doing math and using language. It controls the right side of the body, which is usually the action-oriented side.

In general, the right hemisphere is the sensory, intuitive side. It directs nonverbal activities, such as recognizing faces, visualizing the shape of a pyramid, and responding to music. It controls the left side of the body.

The corpus callosum (Latin for "hard-skinned body"), a bundle of billions of nerve fibers, connects the hemispheres. This neural highway carries messages back and forth, and integrates the memories, perceptions, and responses that each hemisphere processes separately. Thus, our right hemisphere creates an original thought or tune, and our left lets us write it down. Our right and left eyes look at someone and see a whole person, not two separate halves. Our right hand knows what our left hand is doing.

FOUR MAJOR CORTICAL LOBES

Each hemisphere has its own set of four major cortical lobes. Each lobe has a right side and a left side, both of which must work together, relaying neural messages back and forth, in order for the complex task of specialization to occur. The lobes have many administrative duties.

The occipital lobes are for vision. They begin to process visual images before sending them to the parietal and temporal lobes for further interpretation.

The parietal lobes are for body sense. They process proprioceptive messages, so we sense the position of our body in space, and tactile messages such as pain, temperature, and touch discrimination. These lobes interact with other brain parts to give the "whole picture." For instance, they receive visual messages from the occipital lobes and integrate them with auditory and tactile messages, thus aiding vision and spatial awareness.

The Left Hemisphere, Showing the Cortical Lobes, Sensory Cortex, and Motor Cortex

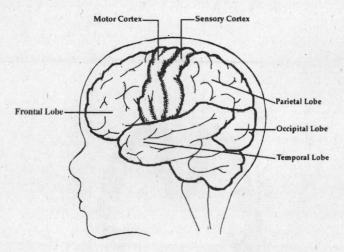

The temporal lobes are for hearing, for interpreting music and language, for refining vestibular sensations, and for memory.

The frontal lobes are for executive thinking. They have a motor area for organizing voluntary body movement, and a prefrontal area concerned with aspects of personality—speech, reasoning, remembering, self-control, problem solving, and planning ahead.

THE SENSORY CORTEX AND
THE MOTOR CORTEX

Lying on the top are strips called the sensory cortex and motor cortex. The sensory cortex receives tactile and proprioceptive sensations from the body. The motor cortex sends messages through peripheral nerves to the muscles.

In the early twentieth century, a Canadian neurosurgeon, Wilder Penfield, studied these cortical areas to learn about neural functions. The "maps" below, based on his research, seem comically out of proportion. Their purpose is serious, however: to illustrate the relative importance of our body parts.

Considerable portions of the sensory cortex are dedicated to receiving messages from the head and the hands—more than from the torso or arm, for instance. The reason is that body function is more important than body size; the head and hands have the most complex functions and thus produce the most sensations. Similarly

Penfield's Maps

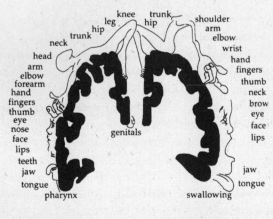

The Sensory Cortex   The Motor Cortex

*Illustrating how the sensory cortex and motor cortex assign specific areas to
different body parts, according to their relative importance.*

large portions of the motor cortex are devoted to sending messages to direct the functions of the fingers, hands, tongue, and throat.

CEREBRAL HEMISPHERES MAKE US HUMAN

Our cerebral hemispheres permit us to learn human skills, such as the ability to stand upright, thereby freeing our hands for manipulating and carrying objects. They enable us to speak, to reason, and to use symbols, thus enabling humankind to develop culture. They allow us to remember the past and to plan for the future, thereby increasing our chances for survival. They give us the mental tools not only to react but also to "pro-act," that is, to anticipate what will happen next and to prepare an appropriate response. The locus of our finest movements and loftiest thoughts, they make us human.

THREE EXAMPLES OF HOW THE CENTRAL NERVOUS SYSTEM PROCESSES SENSATIONS

The Paper Cut

Working at the copy machine, you get a paper cut on your finger. Tactile receptors in your skin send the message via myelinated sensory neurons through your peripheral nervous system to your brain: up your arm, through your spinal cord to your brain stem, to your thalamus, to the sensory cortex. The sensory cortex analyzes the message and tells neurotransmitters to fire excitatory impulses.

First you become aware of the sense of light-touch pressure; a millisecond later, you are conscious of the tissue-damaging pain. Meanwhile, motor neurons send impulses to your finger. You say "Ouch!" and pull your finger away from the paper.

The Fall from the Ladder

Perched on a ladder, you stretch to paint the ceiling. Your triune brain is totally involved: cerebrum, as you plan the next stroke; limbic system, as you smell the paint and remember your first painting experience with Dad; and reptilian complex, as you improve your "nest."

You tilt your chin up a little higher, and your inner ear sends messages to your brain stem about this change of neck and head position. The brain stem relays the vestibular information to your cerebellum, basal ganglia, thalamus, and cerebrum.

Suddenly you feel dizzy, because your head is far off-center. You lose your balance, drop the paint can, and tumble to the floor.

Your hypothalamus registers that you are hurt, afraid, and angry. It alerts your autonomic nervous system to increase your heart rate and to sweat.

You lie in a heap. You can't think about the spilling paint; when you feel endangered, your cerebrum shuts down and the reptilian brain takes over. Your instinct is self-preservation, so you wait until your reticular core calms you down. Regaining control, you realize that you are bruised but not broken. You arise and get busy.

The Car Door Maneuver

Your arms are full of packages and you must close the car door. Your parietal and occipital lobes exchange information to help you gauge your spatial relationship to the car and to plan and execute the maneuver.

Motor neurons send messages through your cerebellum and spinal cord to muscles in your right leg. Excitatory neurons activate muscles on the back of your thigh, instructing them to flex. Inhibitory neurons activate muscles on the front of your thigh, instructing them to extend. Motor planning enables you to bend your knee and lift your right leg.

Meanwhile, the opposite happens in your left leg, which straightens. You stabilize your body and keep your balance.

Proprioceptors in your legs tell your brain what's happening. You push your right foot against the car door and slam it shut.

THE SENSORY PROCESSING MACHINE: SUMMARY

This discussion of the "sensory processing machine" demonstrates the crucial interrelationship of the central nervous system and the senses. It also shows that all parts of the central nervous system must communicate in order to process senses.

It is critical to understand that no matter how much advanced brain power a child has, intelligence alone is not sufficient for organized, daily functioning if the underlying senses are not in good working order. A child's smooth development depends on smooth sensory processing.

APPENDIX B: DR. AYRES'S FOUR
LEVELS OF SENSORY INTEGRATION

In her 1979 book, *Sensory Integration and the Child*, Dr. Ayres described the development of functional skills as "Four Levels of Integration." As you read this summary, please refer to the building blocks illustration on page 67.

LEVEL ONE
(PRIMARY SENSORY SYSTEMS)

The infant busily takes in sensory information, establishing the foundation for all future learning. While the visual, auditory, and other senses are operating, the primary "teachers" are skin (the tactile sense), gravity and movement (the vestibular sense), and muscles (the proprioceptive sense).

Touch stimulation feels good on his skin and around his mouth (an extremely sensitive tactile receptor). He sucks with pleasure and enjoys being held and rocked. A strong feeling of attachment develops as a result of this sensory connection between mother and child. The baby learns that eating, cuddling, and being friendly provide positive feedback.

Through his vestibular and proprioceptive senses, the baby receives information about his movement. He begins to regulate his eye movements, too. He blinks when a speck of dust approaches his eye. With his budding visual sense, he can see motionless objects nearby, as well as people and things moving around him. He anticipates and imitates his mother's facial expressions. He learns to rely on the comings and goings of the people near him.

Vestibular and proprioceptive senses also affect his posture and muscle tone. He tries new movements and, after some effort, succeeds. He lifts his head against gravity, then his shoulders, and, arching up with his weight on his hands and abdomen, he pivots on his stomach and looks around. He hears Mommy sing his name and turns to greet her. Moving in response to the environment is effective. The more he moves, the more confident he becomes.

Vestibular sensations about gravity, coming through his inner ear, teach him that he is connected to the earth. He feels safe.

LEVEL TWO (SENSORY-MOTOR SKILLS)

Having processed basic senses at Level One, the toddler begins to develop body awareness. This is a mental picture of where body parts are, how they interrelate, and how they move. Visual feedback adds to a sense of self.

Along with body awareness comes bilateral (two-sided) integration. This is the process that enables the child to use both sides of his body symmetrically, in a smooth, simultaneous, and coordinated way.

Bilateral integration, a neurological process, is the foundation for bilateral coordination, a behavioral skill. Bilateral coordination is necessary for such interesting work as passing a rattle back and forth from hand to hand.

A function of bilateral integration is lateralization, the process of establishing preference of one side of the brain for directing efficient movement on the opposite side of the body. As lateralization matures, the child begins to demonstrate a hand preference, uses his hands separately, and crosses the midline.

Postural responses improve. The child can get into and stay in different positions. He develops neck stability and can raise his head and torso to look around.

Neck stability helps the eyes hold steady so the child can gaze at whatever interests him. In turn, stabilization of the eyes helps the child improve motor control, for the more he uses his eyes to observe his surroundings, the more he coordinates his movements. With developing binocularity, or eye teaming, he looks where he is going and goes where he is looking.

He begins to crawl, then creep. As he alternates his hands and legs, he uses both sides of his brain and stimulates bilateral coordination.

His maturing tactile, vestibular, and proprioceptive senses promote praxis, or motor planning. He can figure out how to do something he has never done before, and then do it again. Rolling over, for example, requires motor planning the first few times, until the child has practiced it so often that he can roll over effortlessly.

Practicing sensory-motor skills all day long means that the child's activity level becomes better regulated. His attention span and emotional security increase because his sensations are becoming well organized. He can sit in his car seat for a ride to the grocery store. He can bang on the piano keys for a few minutes. He can fall asleep peacefully at the end of his busy day.

LEVEL THREE

(PERCEPTUAL-MOTOR SKILLS)

As the child develops, so does cognitive understanding of the information that his senses take in. As sensory discrimination improves, his ability to interact with the external world broadens.

Hearing (the auditory sense) becomes more refined. He can understand language and communicate through speech.

Vision becomes more precise. He can interpret visual data more accurately. He understands spatial relationships and can discriminate where people and objects are and where he is in relation to them.

Eye-hand coordination develops. Now the child can hold a crayon, draw a simple picture, catch a ball, and pour juice. Eye-hand coordination contributes to visual-motor integration, necessary for such tasks as putting together a string of pop beads, or fitting a jigsaw puzzle piece into place.

Indeed, the child can do a jigsaw puzzle now—just for the fun of it—with purposeful, playful activity. When he picks up a jigsaw piece, it is his developing sensory processing that lets him see it, handle it, understand it, and fit it into the puzzle.

As a preschooler, the child continues to develop and strengthen basic skills. Now he is ready for the top block—the end products of sensory processing, on Level Four.

LEVEL FOUR (ACADEMIC READINESS)

The end products of sensory integration are academic skills (including abstract thought and reasoning), complex motor skills, regulation of attention, organization of behavior, specialization of each side of the body and the brain, visualization, self-esteem, and self-control.

These abilities become increasingly sophisticated. By kindergarten or first grade, the child's brain is mature enough to specialize. Specialization (the process whereby one brain part becomes most efficient at a particular function) means that the child becomes more efficient and purposeful in his actions. His eyes and ears are prepared to take over as the primary "teachers."

He can suppress reflexive responses to unexpected touch

sensations and his tactile discrimination improves. Outdoors on a wintry day, he can ignore the minor discomfort of an itchy wool hat and concentrate on making a snowball. He can tell the difference between a friendly pat and an aggressive punch.

His proprioceptive sense, in tandem with his vestibular and tactile senses, strengthen his motor coordination. His gross-motor skills are smooth: He can jump and run and play with his pals.

His fine-motor skills are good: He can button, zip, and spin a top. He consistently prefers to use one hand more than the other for tool use. He controls a pencil or crayon to make recognizable shapes and symbols.

He can visualize past and future situations: yesterday's ball game and tonight's bath. Visualization helps him picture pretend and real images: make-believe monsters and Mommy's reassuring face.

He is socially competent, able to share ideas and toys, to be flexible when things don't go his way, to empathize with others when things don't go their way, to play by the rules, to be a reliable friend.

The child will continue to process sensations throughout his life. As he encounters different situations and new challenges, he learns to make adaptations in meaningful ways. Feeling good about himself, he is ready for school and the big world.

GLOSSARY

Academic learning: The development of conceptual skills, such as learning to read words and multiply numbers, and to apply what one learns today to what one learned yesterday.

Accommodation: The basic visual skill of focusing on objects at varying distances.

Active touch: Using one's hands, feet, and mouth to gather tactile information about objects in the environment.

Activity level: The degree of one's mental, emotional, or physical arousal. Activity level can be high, low, or in between.

Acuity: The keen perception of a sight, sound or other sensation.

Adaptive behavior: The ability to respond actively and purposefully to changing circumstances and new sensory experiences.

Amygdala: The brain structure that processes smell sensations and produces memories with an emotional component.

Arousal: A state of the nervous system ranging from sleep to awake, from low to high. The optimal state of arousal is the "just right" midpoint between boredom and anxiety, where we feel alert and calm.

Articulation: The production of speech sounds.

Attention-Deficit/Hyperactivity Disorder (ADHD): An umbrella term for a problem interfering with one's ability to attend to and stay focused on meaningful tasks, control one's impulses, and regulate one's activity level. The main symptoms of this neurologically based disorder are hyperactivity, inattention (distractibility), and/or impulsivity.

Audition: The ability to receive and apprehend sounds; hearing.

Auditory discrimination: The ability to receive, identify, differentiate, understand, and respond to sounds.

    Association—Relating novel sound to familiar sound.

    Attention—Maintaining focus sufficiently to listen to voices and sounds.

    Cohesion—Uniting various ideas into a coherent whole and drawing inferences from what is said.

    Discrimination—Differentiating among sounds.

    Figure-ground—Distinguishing between sounds in the foreground and background.

    Localization—Identifying the source of a sound.

    Memory—Remembering what was said.

    Sequencing—Putting what was heard in order.

    Tracking—Following a sound as it moves.

Auditory training: A method of sound stimulation designed to improve a person's listening and communicative skills, learning capabilities, motor coordination, body awareness, and self-esteem.

Autism: A lifelong neurological disability, usually appearing during the first three years of life, which severely impairs the person's sensory processing, verbal and nonverbal communication, social interaction, imagination, problem-solving, and development.

Autonomic nervous system: One of the three components of the nervous system; controls automatic, unconscious bodily functions, such as breathing, sweating, shivering, and digesting.

Aversive response: A feeling of revulsion and repugnance toward a sensation, accompanied by an intense desire to avoid or turn away from it.

Axon: A long fiber extending from the cell body of a neuron that carries impulses away from it to other neurons.

Basal ganglia: The cluster of nerves in the brain that helps coordinate and modulate body movement.

Basic visual skills: Unconscious mechanisms of sight.

Behavior: Whatever one does, through actions, feelings, perceptions, thoughts, words, or movements, in response to stimulation.

Bilateral coordination: The ability to use both sides of the body together in a smooth and simultaneous manner.

Bilateral integration: The neurological process of integrating sensations from both body sides; the foundation for bilateral coordination.

Binocularity (binocular vision; eye teaming): The basic eye-motor skill of forming a single visual image from two images that the eyes separately record.

Bipolar Disorder: An illness involving mood shifts from high to low that affects perceptions, emotions, and behavior; probably caused by dysfunctioning electrical and chemical elements in the brain.

Body awareness, body percept, or **body scheme:** The mental picture of one's own body parts, where they are, how they interrelate, and how they move.

Body position: The placement of one's head, limbs, and trunk. Proprioception is the sense of body position.

Brain: The portion of the CNS that receives sensory messages; integrates, modulates and organizes them; and sends out messages to produce motor, language, or emotional responses.

Brain-behavior: Pertaining to the relationship of incoming sensory messages and outgoing motor, language, or emotional responses.

Brain stem: A primitive brain part, which regulates elementary sensory-motor processes, such as breathing, swallowing, becoming aroused, and calming down.

Central nervous system (CNS): The part of the nervous system, consisting of the brain and spinal cord, that coordinates the activity of the entire nervous system.

Cerebellum: The brain part that directs accurate body movements and balance and processes all other types of sensation.

Cerebral cortex: The outer layer of the cerebrum that coordinates higher nervous activity; also **neocortex**.

Cerebral hemispheres: The two halves of the cerebrum, which continue sensory processing begun at lower levels of the CNS and direct voluntary behavior.

Cerebrum: The front part of the brain where detailed processing of sensations occurs; the "thinking brain."

Compressed visual attention: Focusing on just one object at a time rather than seeing the whole picture.

Cortical lobes: The four sections of the cerebral hemispheres devoted to processing vision, touch, proprioception, memory, hearing, speech, problem solving, voluntary movement, and emotions.

Crossing the midline: Using a hand, foot or eye on the opposite side of the body.

Deep pressure (see **Touch pressure**).

Defensive (or **protective**) **system:** The component of a sensory system that alerts one to real or potential danger and causes a self-protective response. This system is innate.

Developmental delay: The acquisition of specific skills after the expected age.

Diencephalon: The brain part serving as a relay station for incoming sensory information and outgoing motor responses.

Discriminative system: The component of a sensory system that allows one to distinguish differences among and between stimuli. This system is not innate but develops with time and practice.

Distractibility: The inability to fix one's attention on any one stimulus.

Down Syndrome: A congenital disorder, caused by an extra chromosome, that alters the typical development of the brain and body, causing mental retardation.

Dysfunction in sensory integration (DSI): (see **Sensory Processing Disorder**.)

Dyslexia: Severe difficulty in using or understanding language while listening, speaking, reading, writing, or spelling.

Dyspraxia: Difficulty in conceptualizing, motor planning, sequencing, and carrying out unfamiliar actions in a skillful manner. (see **Praxis**.)

Early intervention: Treatment or therapy to prevent problems or to improve a young child's health and development, such as eyeglasses or ear tubes for medical problems, and speech/language therapy or occupational therapy for developmental problems.

Emotional security: The sense that one is lovable and loved, that other people are trustworthy, and that one has the competence to function effectively in everyday life.

Enuresis: Involuntary urination in a child five years or older when no physical abnormality exists.

Essential fatty acids: Substances from fats that must be provided by foods because the body cannot make them, and yet must have them for health.

Evaluation: The use of assessment tools, such as tests and observations, to measure a person's developmental level and individual skills, or to identify a possible difficulty.

Excitation: The neurological process of activating incoming sensory receptors to promote connections between sensory input and behavioral output.

Expressive language: The spoken or written words and phrases that one produces to communicate feelings and thoughts to others.

Extension: The pull of the muscles away from the front of the body; straightening or stretching.

External senses: The senses of touch, smell, taste, vision and hearing; the environmental senses.

Exteroception: Referring to the five external senses.

Eye-hand coordination: The efficient teamwork of the eyes and hands, necessary for activities such as playing with toys, dressing, and writing.

Eye-motor skills—Movements of muscles in the eyes; also **ocular-motor skills**.

> **Fixation**—Steady attention on an object.
> **Saccades**—Efficient movement of the eyes from point to point.
> **Focusing**—Accommodating one's vision smoothly between near and distant objects.
> **Smooth pursuits (tracking)**—Following a moving object or line of print with the eyes.

Far senses: The external or environmental senses of vision and hearing.

Fetal Alcohol Syndrome: A set of symptoms, including growth retardation, facial abnormalities, mental retardation and developmental delays, caused by the mother's chronic alcoholism during pregnancy.

Fight-or-flight response (or **fight-flight-freeze-fright response**): The instinctive reaction to defend oneself from real or perceived danger by becoming aggressive, withdrawing, or being unable to move.

Fine-motor: Referring to movement of the small muscles in the fingers, toes, eyes, and tongue.

Fixing: Pressing one's elbows into one's sides or one's knees together for more stability.

Flexion: Movement of the muscles around a joint to pull a body part toward its front or center; bending.

Floortime: Stanley I. Greenspan's method that fosters children's healthy emotional development through intensive, one-on-one interactions with adults on the child's level.

Fluctuating responsivity: A combination of overresponsivity and underresponsivity as the child's brain rapidly shifts back and forth.

Force (see **Grading of movement**).

Four Fs: Robert Ornstein's way to remember the reflexive, instinctive functions of the limbic system—feeding, fighting, fleeing, and sexual reproduction.

Four Levels: Dr. Ayres' concept of the smooth, sequential development of sensory integration, from infancy through elementary school age.

Fragile X Syndrome: A set of symptoms, including mental retardation, facial anomalies, and deficits in communicative, behavioral, social, and motor skills; caused by an abnormality of the X chromosome.

Grading of movement (force): The ability to flex and extend muscles according to how much pressure is necessary to exert; a function of proprioception.

Gravitational insecurity: Extreme fear and anxiety that one will fall when one's head position changes or when moving through space, resulting from poor vestibular and proprioceptive processing.

Gravity receptors: Organs in the inner ear that respond to changes in gravitational pull.

Gross motor: Referring to movement of large muscles in the arms, legs, and trunk.

Gustatory sense: The sense of perceiving flavor; taste.

Habituation: The neurological process of tuning out familiar sensations.

Hand preference: Right- or lefthandedness, which becomes established as lateralization develops in the brain.

Hidden senses: Internal senses.

Hippocampus: The brain part that compares old and new sensory stimuli and is involved with memory.

Hyperactivity: Excessive mobility, motor function, or activity, such as fingertapping, jumping from one's seat, or constantly moving some part of the body; "fidgetiness."

Hypersensitivity, Hyperreactivity, Overresponsiveness (see **Overresponsivity**).

Hyposensitivity, Hyporeactivity, Hyporesponsiveness (see **Underresponsivity**).

Hypothalamus: The brain structure that regulates unconscious bodily processes such as body temperature and metabolic functions.

IDEA: The Individuals with Disabilities Education Act, P.L. 99–457, and amendments. This legislation requires school districts to provide occupational therapy as a related service to children who need it in order to benefit from education.

Ideation: The process of forming or conceiving of an action to take; the first step in **Praxis.**

IEP: Individualized Education Program, a legal document specifying the needs of a child identified as having a disability and providing for special education and related services.

Impulse control: Difficulty in restraining one's actions, words, or emotions.

Increased tolerance for movement: Underresponsivity to typical amounts of movement stimulation; often characterized by craving for intense movement experiences such as rocking and spinning.

Inhibition: The neurological process that checks one's overreaction to sensations.

Inner drive: Every person's self-motivation to participate actively in experiences that promote sensory processing.

Inner ear: The organ that receives sensations of the pull of gravity and of changes in balance and head position.

Integration: The combination of many parts into a unified, harmonious whole.

"Internal eyes": Body awareness.

Internal senses: The subconscious senses that regulate bodily functions, such as heart rate, hunger, and arousal, including the interoceptive, vestibular, and proprioceptive senses. Also called the **hidden, special, near,** or **somatosensory senses**.

Interoception: The body-centered sense involving both the conscious awareness and the unconscious regulation of bodily processes of the heart, liver, stomach, and other internal organs.

Intersensory integration: The convergence of sensations of touch, body position, movement, sight, sound, and smell.

Intolerance to movement: The overreactivity to moving or being moved rapidly, often characterized by extreme distress when spinning or by avoidance of movement through space.

Kinesthesia: The conscious awareness of joint position and body movement in space, such as knowing where to place one's feet when climbing stairs, without visual cues.

Language: The organized use of words and phrases to interpret what one hears or reads and to communicate one's thoughts and feelings.

Lateralization: The process of establishing preference of one side of the brain for directing skilled motor function on the opposite side of the body, while the opposite body side is used for stabilization; necessary for hand preference and crossing the midline.

Learned helplessness: The tendency to depend on others for guidance and decisions, to lack self-help skills, and to be a passive learner; often related to poor self-esteem.

Learning disability: An identified difficulty with reading, writing, spelling, computing, and communicating. (SPD may cause significant learning problems that are often neither recognized nor identified as learning disabilities.)

Light touch (see **Touch pressure**).

Limbic system: The brain part that processes messages from all the senses and is involved primarily with emotions and inner drive; the "seat of emotions"; the "smell brain."

Linear movement: A motion in which one moves in a line, from front to back, side to side, or up and down.

Low tone (see **Muscle tone**).

Meltdown: The process, usually caused by excessive sensory stimulation, of becoming "undone" or "unglued," accompanied by screaming, writhing, and deep sobbing.

Mental retardation: Significantly subaverage intellectual functioning and impairments in adaptive behavior; caused by injury, disease, or abnormality before age eighteen.

Midline: A median line dividing the two halves of the body. (See **Crossing the midline**.)

Modulation: The brain's ability to regulate and organize the degree, intensity, and nature of the person's response to sensory input in a graded and adaptive manner.

Motor control: The ability to regulate and monitor the motions of one's muscles for coordinated movement.

Motor coordination: The ability of several muscles or muscle groups to work together harmoniously to perform movements.

Motor cortex: The portion of the cerebrum that sends out messages to direct the movement and coordination of muscles; also **motor strip**.

Motor learning: The process of mastering simple movement skills essential for developing more complex movement skills.

Motor planning: The ability to organize and sequence the steps of an unfamiliar and complex body movement in a coordinated manner; a piece of praxis.

Muscle tone: The degree of tension normally present when one's muscles are relaxed, or in a resting state; a function of the vestibular system, enabling the person to maintain body position. **Low tone** is the lack of supportive muscle tone, usually with increased mobility at the joints; the person with low tone seems "loose and floppy."

Myelination: The gradual insulation of a neural axon with a fatty substance called myelin.

Neurology: The science of the nerves and the nervous system. A **neurologist** is a physician who diagnoses and treats diseases of the brain and central nervous system, but usually not SPD.

Neuromuscular: Relating to the relationship of nerves and muscles.

Neuron: The nerve cell, which is the functional and structural unit of the nervous system and the fundamental building block of the brain. **Sensory neurons** receive messages from receptors in the eyes, ears, skin, muscles, joints, and organs; and **motor neurons** send out messages to the body for appropriate responses.

Obsessive-Compulsive Disorder (OCD): An anxiety disorder marked by recurrent, persistent, inappropriate thoughts and by repetitive behaviors such as hand washing.

Occupational therapy (OT): The use of activity to maximize the independence and the maintenance of health of an individual who is limited by a physical injury or illness, cognitive impairment, psychosocial dysfunction, mental illness, developmental or learning disability, or adverse environmental condition. OT encompasses evaluation, assessment, treatment, and consultation. An **occupational therapist** (also **OT**) is a health professional trained in the biological, physical, medical, and behavioral sciences, including neurology, anatomy, development, kinesiology, orthopedics, psychiatry, and psychology.

Ocular-motor (see **Eye-motor skills**).

Olfactory sense: The far sense that perceives odor; smell.

Optometrist or **Developmental optometrist:** A specialist who examines eyes, prescribes lenses, and provides vision therapy to prevent or eliminate visual problems and enhance a person's visual performance.

Oral apraxia: A sensory-based motor problem affecting the ability to produce and sequence sounds necessary for speech.

Oral defensiveness: Overresponsivity in the mouth to certain food textures or tastes.

Oral-motor skills: Movements of muscles in the mouth, lips, tongue, and jaw, including sucking, biting, crunching, chewing, and licking.

Oscillation: Up-and-down or to-and-fro linear movement, such as swinging, bouncing, and jumping.

Overreactivity and Underreactivity: Exaggerated neurological and physiological processes that we cannot observe and that may cause over- and underresponsive behavior.

Overresponsivity: Observable behavior involving a quick or intense response to sensory stimuli that others usually perceive as benign; characterized by exaggerated, negative, and emotional responses (fight-or-flight) or withdrawal (flight or freeze).

Passive movement: The act of being moved by something or someone.

Passive touch: The act of being touched by something or someone without initiating it.

Perception: The meaning that the brain gives to sensory input.

Peripheral nervous system (PNS): One of the three components of the nervous system. Through the spinal cord, peripheral nerves in one's skin, eyes, ears, muscles, and organs send sensory impulses to the brain and receive motor impulses from the brain.

Pervasive Developmental Disorder: Severe, overall impairment in the ability to regulate sensory experiences, affecting the child's affect and behavior, interaction with others, and communication skills; similar to, but milder than, autism.

Physical therapy: A health profession devoted to improving one's physical abilities through activities that strengthen muscular control and motor coordination, especially of the large muscles.

Plasticity: The ability of the brain to change or to be changed as a result of activity, especially as one responds to sensations.

Postural background adjustments: Automatic movements in one's trunk and limbs, allowing a person to use only the muscles necessary for a particular motion.

Postural Disorder: Difficulty with moving or stabilizing the body to meet the demands of the environment or a particular motor task.

Postural stability: The feeling of security and self-confidence when moving in space, based on one's body awareness. SPD may cause **postural insecurity**, the feeling that one's body is not stable.

Praxis: The ability to interact successfully with the physical environment; to ideate, plan, organize, and carry out a sequence of unfamiliar actions; and to do what one needs and wants to do. **Praxis** (Greek for "doing, action, practice") is a broad term denoting voluntary and coordinated action. **Motor planning** is often used as a synonym.

Prefrontal cortex: The cortical lobe in the brain that coordinates speech, reasoning, remembering, problem solving, self-control, and planning ahead.

Proprioception/Proprioceptive sense (the position sense): The unconscious awareness of sensations coming from one's muscles and joints that provides information about when and how muscles contract or stretch; when and how joints bend, extend, or are pulled; and where each part of the body is and how it is moving.

Protective extension: Thrusting out an arm or leg to protect oneself while falling.

Protective system (see **Defensive system**).

Psychotherapy: Treatment by psychological means of mental, emotional, or behavior problems.

Receptive language: The ability to understand how words express ideas and feelings; language that one takes in by listening and reading.

Receptors: Special cells, located throughout one's body, which receive specific sensory messages and send them for processing to the CNS.

Reflex: An automatic, innate response to sensory stimulation.

Regulatory disorder: A problem with adapting to changing conditions, such as self-calming when distressed; falling asleep and waking up; eating, digesting, and eliminating; paying attention; participating socially; and processing sensations.

Reptilian brain: In evolutionary terms, the oldest part of the brain, controlling reflexive, instinctive behavior; the "primitive brain."

Reticular core: A network of neurons in the brain stem that receives impulses from every sensory system and is the center for arousal and for calming down.

Rotary movement: Turning or spinning in circles.

Satiety: Fullness.

Screening: A quick, informal procedure for the early identification of children's health or developmental problems.

Selective mutism: A childhood anxiety disorder characterized by the inability to speak and communicate comfortably in select social settings.

Self-help skills: Competence in taking care of one's personal needs, such as bathing, dressing, eating, grooming, and studying.

Self-regulation: The ability to control one's activity level and state of alertness, as well as one's emotional, mental, or physical responses to sensations; self-organization.

Self-therapy: Active, voluntary participation in experiences that promote self-regulation, such as spinning in circles to stimulate one's vestibular system.

Sensitization: The process of interpreting stimuli as important, unfamiliar, or harmful, even if the stimuli are unimportant, familiar, and benign.

Sensory-Based Motor Disorder: A problem with movement, such as **Postural Disorder** and **Dyspraxia**, resulting from inefficient sensory processing.

Sensory cortex: The portion of the cerebrum that receives sensations from the body; also **sensory strip**.

Sensory defensiveness: The tendency to respond to certain harmless sensations as if they were dangerous or painful; also **overresponsivity.**

Sensory diet: The multisensory experiences that one normally seeks on a daily basis to satisfy one's sensory appetite; a planned and scheduled activity program that an occupational therapist develops to help a person become more self-regulated.

Sensory Discrimination Disorder: Problems in discerning the characteristics of sensory stimuli and the differences among and between stimuli.

Sensory integration (SI): The part of sensory processing whereby sensations from one or more sensory systems connect in the brain. SI dysfunction is another term for SPD.

Sensory integration theory: A concept based on neurology, research, and behavior that explains the brain-behavior relationship.

Sensory integration treatment: A technique of occupational therapy, which provides playful, meaningful activities that enhance an individual's sensory intake and lead to more adaptive functioning in daily life. The emphasis is on improving sensory-motor processing rather than on skill training.

Sensory Modulation Disorder: The inability to regulate and organize the degree, intensity, and nature of responses to sensory input in a graded and adaptive manner.

Sensory-motor: Pertaining to the brain-behavior process of taking in sensory messages and reacting with a physical response.

Sensory Processing Disorder (SPD): Difficulty in the way the brain takes in, organizes and uses sensory information, causing a person to have problems interacting effectively in the everyday environment. Sensory stimulation may cause difficulty in one's movement, emotions, attention, relationships, or adaptive responses.

"Sensory processing machine": Dr. A. Jean Ayres's term for the brain.

Sensory seeking: The constant quest for excessive sensory stimulation.

Sequencing: Putting movements, sounds, sights, objects, thoughts, letters, and numbers in consecutive order, according to time and space.

Sleep regulation problem: An irregular pattern of sleeping, such as difficulty falling asleep or sleeping through the night, or the need for an unusual amount of sleep.

Social skills: Effective interaction and communication with others, necessary for developing and keeping friendships.

Somatosensory: Referring to tactile-proprioceptive discrimination of touch sensations and body position; body sensing.

Special education: Individualized instruction for the child who has difficulty learning at school.

Specialization: The process whereby one part of the brain becomes most efficient at a particular function.

Speech: The physical act of communicating a verbal message.

Speech-and-language therapy: Treatment to help a person develop or improve articulation, communication skills, and oral-motor skills.

Spinal cord: The long, thick cord of nervous tissue that receives tactile and proprioceptive messages from skin, joints, and muscles, and that sends out motor messages for movement.

Splinter skill: An isolated ability that one develops with much effort, but that one cannot generalize for other purposes.

State: The degree of one's attentiveness, mood, or motor response to sensory stimulation.

Stereotypical behavior: Nonproductive, repetitive, and habitual actions often associated with autism.

Stimulus (pl., stimuli): Something that activates a sensory receptor and produces a response.

Synapse: The junction of two neurons where an impulse is transmitted from one to another.

Syndrome: A group of unrelated characteristics varying in severity from one individual to another, such as **Asperger Syndrome** or **dyslexia**.

Tactile defensiveness: The tendency to react negatively and emotionally to unexpected, light-touch sensations; a common type of sensory modulation dysfunction.

Tactile discrimination: The awareness of touching or of being touched by something; the ability to distinguish differences in touch sensations; and the awareness of the physical attributes of an object, such as its size, shape, temperature, density, and texture.

Tactile-proprioceptive: Referring to simultaneous sensations of touch and body position.

Tactile sense (the sense of touch): The sensory system that receives sensations of pressure, vibration, movement, temperature, and pain, primarily through receptors in the skin and hair. Protective receptors respond to light or unexpected touch and help a person avoid bodily harm; discriminative receptors provide information about the tactile qualities of the object or person being touched.

Thalamus: The brain part that processes all sensations except smell.

Touch pressure: The tactile stimulus that causes receptors in the skin to respond. **Deep pressure**, such as a hug, activates receptors in the discriminative system. **Light touch**, such as a kiss, activates receptors in the protective system.

Triune brain: Paul MacLean's theory that the brain is composed of three systems (the reptilian complex, the limbic system, and the cerebrum).

Underresponsivity: Undersensitivity to sensory stimuli, characterized by a tendency either to crave intense sensations or to withdraw and be difficult to engage; a subtype of sensory modulation disorder.

Unilateral coordination: Smooth, independent use of one side of the body, necessary for writing and handling tools.

Vestibular sense (the balance and movement sense): The sensory system that responds to the pull of gravity, providing information about the head's position in relation to the surface of the earth, and coordinating movements of the eyes, head, and body that affect equilibrium, muscle tone, vision, hearing, and emotional security. Receptors are in the inner ear.

Vestibular-proprioceptive: Referring to simultaneous sensations of head and body position when one moves.

Vision: The process of identifying sights, understanding what the eyes see, and preparing for a response.

Vision therapy: Treatment to help a person improve visual skills and to prevent learning-related visual problems; optometric visual training.

Visualization: The act of forming mental images of objects, people, or scenarios.

Visual discrimination: The ability to perceive and interpret sensory information received through the eyes and body as one interacts with the environment and moves one's body through space.

Attention—The use of the eyes, brain, and body together long enough to stay with an activity.

Depth perception—The ability to see objects in three dimensions and to judge relative distances between objects, or between oneself and objects.

Discrimination—Discernment of likenesses and differences in size, shape, pattern, form, position, and color.

Figure-ground—Differentiation between objects in the foreground and background.

Form constancy—Recognition of a shape regardless of its size, position, or texture.

Memory—Recognizing, associating, storing and retrieving visual details.

Peripheral vision—Awareness of images through the sides of the eyes.

Position in space—Awareness of the spatial orientation of letters, words, numbers, or drawings on a page, or of an object in the environment.

Sequential memory—Perception of words and pictures in order.

Spatial relationships—Awareness of directionality (how close objects are) and laterality (right/left, front/back, up/down), and how to move around objects.

Stable visual field—Discernment of which objects move and which stay still.

Visual-sensory integration—Combining sights with touch, movement, and other sensory messages.

Visualization—Forming and manipulating images of objects, people or scenes in one's mind's eye.

Visual-motor skills: One's movements based on the discrimination of visual information.

Eye-hand coordination—The eyes' guidance of guide fine-motor tasks.

Eye-foot coordination—The eyes' guidance of gross-motor activities.

Eye-ear coordination—The ability to see a letter or word, and say or use it.

RESOURCES

For updates, please see www.out-of-sync-child.com.

CATALOGS FOR
EQUIPMENT AND MATERIALS

Abilitations

(800) 850-8602   www.abilitations.com

Rehabilitation products designed to improve the lives of children with differing abilities.

Achievement Products for Children

(800) 373-4699   www.specialkidszone.com

Products that make life more comfortable for children with sensory problems.

Future Horizons

(817) 277-0727; or toll-free, (888) 489-0727
www.futurehorizons-autism.com

Publishing and conferences featuring autism, Asperger syndrome, early intervention, etc.

In Your Pocket Designs

(804) 379-0944   www.weightedvest.com

Weighted vests to provide the deep pressure to help some children self-calm and relax.

Integrations

(800) 622-0638   www.integrationscatalog.com

User-friendly product line for kids with learning and sensory differences in various settings, with information tips written in an educator's language.

Mozart Effect® Resource Center

(314) 531-7656; toll-free, (800) 721-2177 www.mozarteffect.com

Books and recordings about the powers of music in health, education, and well-being.

OT Ideas, Inc.

(973) 895-3622   www.otideas.com

Scissors, tools, and toys to develop hand coordination, fine-motor and visual-motor skills.

PDP Products & Professional Development Programs

(651) 439-8865   www.pdppro.com

Materials and conferences that promote sensory processing, attention, and self-regulation.

Playaway Toy Company, Inc.

(715) 752-4565; toll free, (888) PLAYWAY
www.playawaytoy.com

The Rainy Day Indoor Playground and other innovative, fun indoor gym equipment. Interchangeable parts include swings, trapeze bar, glider, net, platform and ladder. Requiring no tools to install, the set is transportable from door to door.

Pocket Full of Therapy, Inc.

(732) 441-0404; toll free, (800) PFOT-124   www.pfot.com

Equipment and fun materials to use to motivate children with special needs.

Sensory Comfort
(603) 436-8797; toll free, (888) 436-2622
www.sensorycomfort. com

Products for adults and children, including seamless socks, to make life more comfortable for those with sensory processing differences.

Sensory Resources, LLC
(702) 433-0404; toll free, (888) 357-5867
www.sensoryresources.com

Resources for raising children with sensory-motor, developmental, and social-emotional challenges. National conferences on sensory processing and related subjects. Publications including *The Out-of-Sync Child* (video), *Getting Kids in Sync* (video), *Teachers Ask About Sensory Integration* (audio), *Answers to Questions Teachers Ask About Sensory Integration* (reference book), *The Goodenoughs Get in Sync* (a "chapter book" for ages 8–12 about five family members with SPD) and *Preschool SENsory Scan for Educators (Preschool SENSE),* a screening tool for OTs to use in schools.

SensoryEdge.com
(818) 788-2434   www.sensoryedge.com

Specializing in children's furniture, rocking chairs, and educational, sensory-based toys.

Southpaw Enterprises
(800) 228-1698   www.southpawenterprises.com

Sensory and developmental products for therapists to use with children with special needs.

Theragifts Sensory Diet Toys and Products
(603) 437-3330   www.theragifts.com

Sensory-motor products, toys, and gifts for children with SPD, autism and other delays.

Therapro
(508) 872-9494; toll free, (800) 257-5376
www.theraproducts.com

Equipment and toys, including unique kits for sensory-motor awareness and skills.

The Therapy Shoppe®, Inc.
(616) 863-5978; toll-free, (800) 261-5590
www.TherapyShoppe. com
    Sensory-motor equipment for use by schools and therapists, parents and teachers.

Therapy Skill Builders
(800) 228-0752   www.psychcorp.com
    Resources for OTs, from widely-used assessments to innovative therapy products.

TherapyWorks, Inc.
(505) 897-3478   www.alertprogram.com
    Products related to *How Does Your Engine Run? The Alert Program for Self-Regulation.*

ORGANIZATIONS

Achievers Unlimited, Inc.
(800) 924-9897   www.achieverswisconsin.org
    Services and materials to improve children's motor and visual development.

American Occupational Therapy Association, Inc. (AOTA)
(301) 652-AOTA; toll free, (800) 729-2682   www.aota.org
    Books, videos, continuing education workshops, and other resources for OTs.

American Speech-Language-Hearing Association (ASHA)
(301) 897-5700; toll free, (800) 638-TALK   www.asha.org
    Printed materials and referrals to local audiologists and speech/language therapists.

Autism Network for Dietary Intervention (ANDI)
www.autismNDI.com
    Support for families using a gluten- and casein-free diet in the treatment of autism.

The Council for Exceptional Children (CEC)
(703) 620-3660; toll free, (888) CEC-SPED   www.cec.sped.org

Federally funded clearinghouse of publications on disabilities—the "voice and vision of special education."

Developmental Delay Resources (DDR)
(412) 422-3373 (PA), or (800)497-0944   www.devdelay.org

Publications, conferences, and quarterly newsletter, *New Developments,* to educate parents and professionals about healthy options for treating the whole child.

Families and Advocates Partnership for Education (FAPE)
www.fape.org

U.S. Dept. of Education project to improve educational outcomes for children with disabilities. FAPE provides parents, administrators, service providers, and policymakers with information about implementing IDEA '04.

Henry Occupational Therapy Services, Inc. (HOTS)
(623) 933-3821; toll free, (888) 371-1204   www.ateachabout.com

Diana Henry's workshops, videos and handbooks for parents, teachers, and students.

KID Foundation (Knowledge In Development Foundation)
(303) 794-1182   www.KIDFoundation and   www.SPDnetwork.org

Public charity that serves children with SPD by increasing awareness of the scope and severity of the disorder; providing information and resources to families and professionals; and supporting research. KID Foundation programs include:

• **Sensory Processing Disorder-Parent Connections**, supporting parents of children with SPD. Run by local hosts nationwide, dozens of chapters provide monthly or quarterly meetings.

• **International Resource Directory**, providing *free* information about physicians, dentists, OTs, PTs, SLPs, eyecare, and mental health professionals, educators, facilities, assessment and intervention.

• **Advocacy for Diagnostic Acceptance**, working toward the inclusion of SPD as a valid diagnosis in existing classification systems, including *Diagnostic and Statistical Manual (DSM-V)*, *International Classification of Diseases (ICD-11)*, and *Diagnostic Classification 0 to 3 (DC: 0–3 Revised and DC: 0–3 II)*.

• **Support of Research**, through fundraising and granting of funds when possible. A primary arm of research is conducted at the Sensory processing Treatment And Research (STAR) Center at The Children's Hospital of Denver (Dr. Lucy Miller, Director).

• **Dissemination of Information**, making available a large variety of *free* online articles and resources, through www. KIDFoundation.org and its companion website, www. SPDnetwork.org

Learning Disabilities Center (LDA)
(412) 341-1515   www.ldanatl.org
Resources for professionals and parents.

National Fragile X Foundation
(925) 938-9300; toll free, (800) 688-8765   http://fragilex.org
Supporting families and research toward improved treatments and cure for this syndrome.

National Information Center for Children and Youth with Disabilities (NICHCY)
(800) 695-0285   www.nichcy.org
Clearinghouse for families, professionals, educators, and others working with disability-related issues, including fact sheets on IDEA and legal aspects of education.

Nonverbal Learning Disorders Association (NLDA)
East Coast: (860) 693-3738 West Coast: (925) 820-4079
www. NLDline.com
Support for those with impaired reception of nonverbal, performance-based information.

Optometric Extension Program Foundation, Inc.
(949) 250-8070   www.oep.org
Books and materials on vision development, vision therapy, and research in vision.

The Parent Network for The Post-Institutionalized Child (PNPIC)
(724) 222-1776 (voice mail only)   http://pnpic.org
Support for adoptive families of children primarily from Eastern Bloc orphanages.

Parents Active for Vision Education (PAVE)
(619) 287-0081, toll free 800-PAVE-988   www.pavevision.org
Information about the relationship between vision and academic achievement.

Parents/Professionals for Exceptional Progress (PEP)
(225) 755-2304   www.pep-usa.org
Research information on all treatments and care for children who are sensory challenged.

***S.I. FOCUS* Magazine**
c/o Shannon Media, P.O. Box 821404, Dallas, TX 75382
(214) 341-9999   www.SIfocus.com
International, quarterly magazine focusing on sensory integration/sensory processing, filled with success stories, clinical breakthroughs, therapy techniques and in-depth interviews. An online store offers new products, books, clothing, and other special items. (I am editor-in-chief.)

Zero to Three
(202) 638-1144; toll free, (800) 899-4301   www.zerotothree.org
Services, conferences, and publications to improve the physical, cognitive, emotional, and social development of infants, toddlers, and families.

ADDITIONAL INTERNET RESOURCES

In addition to the websites listed above, these may also be helpful:
www.abilitiescenter.com
www.autism.org
www.autismawarenesscentre.com
www.childhoodanxietynetwork.org
www.floortime.org
www.otawatertown.com
www.sensorytools.net
www.vitallinks.net
www.wrightslaw.com

About the Author

Carol Stock Kranowitz, a music, movement, and drama teacher for twenty-five years, observed many out-of-sync preschoolers. To help them become more competent in their work and play, she began to study sensory integration ("SI") theory. She learned to help identify their needs and steer them into early intervention. In her workshops and writings, she explains to parents, educators, and other early childhood professionals how Sensory Processing Disorder plays out—and provides practical and enjoyable techniques for addressing sensory issues at home and school.

A graduate of Barnard College, Carol has an MA in education and human development from The George Washington University. She is the editor-in-chief of *S.I. Focus,* the international magazine focusing on sensory integration/sensory processing. She lives in Bethesda, Maryland, and has two married sons and four enchanting grandchildren.

Carol's publications include:
*The Out-of-Sync Child: Recognizing and Coping with Sensory Processing Disorder, 2*nd *ed.* (Perigee, 2005)

The Out-of-Sync Child Has Fun: Activities for Kids with Sensory Integration Dysfunction (Perigee, 2003)

The Goodenoughs Get in Sync: An Introduction to SPD (Sensory Resources, 2004)

101 Activities for Kids in Tight Spaces (St. Martin's Press, 1995)

Hear, See, Play! Music Discovery Activities for Preschoolers, with Kay Jones (Peg Hoenack's MusicWorks, 1989)

The Balzer-Martin Preschool Screening Program Manual, with Lynn Balzer-Martin, PhD, OTR (St. Columba's, 1992)

The Out-of-Sync Child video (Sensory Resources, 2001)

Getting Kids in Sync: Sensory-Motor Activities to Help Children Develop Body Awareness video (Sensory Resources, 2002)

Teachers Ask about Sensory Integration audiotape, with Stacey Szklut, MS, OTR/L (Sensory Resources, 1999)

Answers to Questions Teachers Ask about Sensory Integration, with Stacey Szklut, et al. (Sensory Resources, 2002)

For more information, visit the Out-of-Sync Child web site, www.out-of-sync-child.com

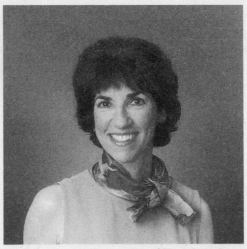

Photo by Beverly Rezneck

SELECTED BIBLIOGRAPHY

AUTISM AND ASPERGER SYNDROME

Autism fact sheet (2003). Bethesda, MD: Office of Communications and Public Liaison, National Institute of Neurological Disorders and Stroke, National Institutes of Health.
www.ninds.nih.gov/health_and_medical/pubs/autism.htm

Grandin, Temple, PhD (1996). *Thinking in Pictures and Other Reports from My Life with Autism.* New York: Vintage.

———— (1999). *Sensory Challenges and Answers* (video). Arlington, TX: Future Horizons.

———— (June 2000). My experiences with visual thinking, sensory problems and communication difficulties.
www.autism.org/temple/visual.html

Greenspan, Stanley I., MD (March 23, 2003). Notes on intervention efficacy for autistic spectrum disorders. E-mail message.

Huebner, Ruth A., PhD, & Winnie Dunn, PhD (2001).

Introduction and basic concepts. In *Autism: A Sensorimotor Approach to Management,* edited by Ruth A. Huebner. Gaithersburg, MD: Aspen Publishers.

Moyes, Rebecca A. (2002). *Addressing the Challenging Behavior of Children with High-Functioning Autism/Asperger Syndrome in the Classroom: A Guide for Teachers and Parents.* London: Jessica Kingsley Pub.

Myles, Brenda Smith, PhD, Katherine Tapscott Cook, Nancy E. Miller, Louann Rinner & Lisa A. Robbins (2000). *Asperger Syndrome and Sensory Issues: Practical Solutions for Making Sense of the World.* Shawnee Mission, KS: Asperger Autism.

Shore, Stephen (2002). *Beyond the Wall: Personal Experiences with Autism and Asperger Syndrome.* Shawnee Mission, KS: Autism Asperger.

——— (Summer 2004). Perception. *S.I. Focus* magazine.

Seroussi, Karyn (2000). *Unraveling the Mystery of Autism and Pervasive Developmental Disorder: A Mother's Story of Research and Recovery.* New York: Simon & Schuster.

Smith, Dr. Ruth (2002). Sensory and motor problems in individuals with Asperger's syndrome. Waltham, MA: The E. K. Shriver Center at the University of Massachusetts Medical School. www.ddleadership.org/aspergers/courses/sensory/

Stacey, Patricia (2003). *The Boy Who Loved Windows: Opening the Heart and Mind of a Child Threatened with Autism.* Cambridge, MA: Da Capo Press.

Waltz, Mitzi (2002). *Autistic Spectrum Disorders: Understanding the Diagnosis and Getting Help.* Sebastopol, CA: O'Reilly & Associates.

THE BRAIN

Berthoz, Alain (2000). *The Brain's Sense of Movement.* Translated by Giselle Weiss. Cambridge, MA: Harvard University Press.

Eliot, Lise, PhD (1999). *What's Going on in There? How the Brain and Mind Develop in the First Five Years of Life*. New York: Bantam.

Healy, Jane M., PhD (1999). *Endangered Minds: Why Children Don't Think—and What We Can Do About It*. New York: Simon & Schuster/Touchstone.

———— (2004). *Your Child's Growing Mind: Brain Development and Learning from Birth to Adolescence* (3rd ed.). New York: Broadway.

———— (Spring 1996). Children's brains at work in the preschool and primary years. *Early Childhood Connections*.

Just, Marcel Adam, PhD, Vladimir L. Cherkassky, PhD, Timothy A. Keller, & Nancy J. Minshew, MD (August 2004). Cortical activation and synchronization during sentence comprehension in high-functioning autism: Evidence of underconnectivity. *Brain*, 127(8).

MacLean, Paul D., PhD (1973). *A Triune Concept of the Brain and Behavior*. Toronto, Canada: University of Toronto.

Ornstein, Robert, & Richard Thompson (1991). *The Amazing Brain*. New York: Mariner. (The "Four Fs.")

Parker, Steve (1990). *The Brain and Nervous System*. New York: Franklin Watts.

Sagan, Carl, PhD (1977). *The Dragons of Eden: Speculations on the Evolution of Human Intelligence*. New York: Random House.

EATING AND NUTRITION

Dorfman, Kelly (Summer 1998). How sensory integration and nutrition interact, *New Developments*, 4(1); (Spring 1999) The picky eater, *New Developments*, 4(4); (Summer 1999) Calming the brain, *New Developments*, 5(1); and (Summer 2003) How the immune system talks to the nervous system, *New Developments*, 8(4). Bethesda, MD: Developmental Delay Resources (DDR).

Ernsperger, Lori, PhD, & Tania Stegen-Hanson (2004). *Just Take a Bite: Easy, Effective Answers to Food Aversions and Eating Challenges!* Arlington, TX: Future Horizons.

Laake, Dana (October 16, 2004). Nutritional approaches. Lecture presented at Special Needs, Special Kids conference, Silver Spring, MD.

Tallmadge, Katherine (September 8, 2004). Have your fill. *The Washington Post*. (About nutrition and the sensation of satiety.)

LEARNING, SCHOOLS, AND SPECIAL EDUCATION

Hannaford, Carla (1995). *Smart Moves: Why Learning Is Not All In Your Head.* Arlington, VA: Great Ocean Publishers.

Furth, Hans G., & Harry Wachs, OD (1982). *Thinking Goes to School: Piaget's Theory in Practice.* New York: Oxford University Press.

Individuals with Disabilities Education Improvement Act of 2004, referred to as *IDEA 04* (Public Law 108–446). http://edworkforce.house.gov/issues/108th/education/idea/conferencereport/confrept.htm

Kay, Kiesa, ed. (2000). *Uniquely Gifted: Identifying and Meeting the Needs of the Twice-Exceptional Student.* Gilsum, NH: Avocus Publishing.

Kranowitz, C.S. (2005). *Preschool SENSE (SENsory Scan for Educators): A Tool for OTs in Schools.* Las Vegas: Sensory Resources.

———, and Stacey Szklut (1999). *Teachers Ask About Sensory Integration* (audiotape). Las Vegas: Sensory Resources.

———, Jane Koomar, PhD, Stacey Szklut, Lynn Balzer-Martin, PhD, Elizabeth Haber, & Deanna Iris Sava (2001). *Answers to Questions Teachers Ask About Sensory Integration Dysfunction.* Las Vegas: Sensory Resources.

Kline, Frank M., PhD, Larry B. Silver, MD, & Steven C. Russell, eds. (2001). *The Educator's Guide to Medical Issues in the Classroom.* Baltimore: Paul H. Brookes. (Particularly pertinent chapters include: Pervasive developmental disorders, by Rosa A. Hagin, PhD; Sensory integration dysfunction, by Lynn A. Balzer-Martin, PhD, and Carol Kranowitz, and Attention-deficit/hyperactivity disorder, by Larry B. Silver, MD.)

Quirk, Norma J., & Marie E. DiMatties (1990). *The Relationship of Learning Problems and Classroom Performance to Sensory Integration.* Cherry Hill, NJ: Author (Norma Quirk, 131 Dumas Rd., 08003).

Sassé, Margaret (1990). *If Only We'd Known . . . Early Childhood—and Its Importance to Academic Learning.* Victoria, Australia: Toddler Kindy Gymbaroo Pty., Ltd.

Schneider, Catherine Chemin (2001). *Sensory Secrets: How to Jump-Start Learning in Children.* Siloam Springs, AR: Concerned Communications.

Shipon-Blum, Elisa, DO (2003). *The Ideal Classroom Setting for the Selectively Mute Child: A Guide for Parents, Teachers and Treating Professionals* (2nd ed.). Philadelphia: Selective Mutism Anxiety Research and Treatment Center.

Shaywitz, Sally, MD (2003). *Overcoming Dyslexia: A New and Complete Science-Based Program for Overcoming Reading Problems at Any Level.* New York: Knopf.

Silver, Larry B., MD (1998). *The Misunderstood Child: Understanding and Coping with Your Child's Learning Disabilities* (3rd ed.). New York: Three Rivers Press.

Smith, Sally L. (1995). *No Easy Answers: The Learning Disabled Child at Home and at School.* New York: Bantam.

Vuko, Evelyn Porreca (2004). *Teacher Says: 30 Foolproof Ways to Help Kids Thrive in School.* New York: Perigee.

Wright, Peter W. D., & Pamela Darr Wright (1999). *Wrightslaw: Special Education Law.* Hartfield, VA: Harbor House Law Press.

LISTENING

AND THE AUDITORY SYSTEM

Burk, Ricky W. (1999). Interview with Dorothy Kelly, DA, CCC-S, about central auditory processing disorder (CAPD). www.mshausa.org/kelly.html.

Campbell, Don (2000). *The Mozart Effect for Children: Awakening Your Child's Mind, Health, and Creativity with Music.* New York: HarperCollins.

Frick, Sheila M., & Colleen Hacker (2001). *Listening with the Whole Body.* Madison, WI: Vital Links.

Madaule, Paul (1994). *When Listening Comes Alive: A Guide to Effective Learning and Communication.* Norval, Ontario, Canada: Moulin Publishing.

Thompson, Billie, PhD, et al. (1998). *Listening Checklist.* (Helps parents identify problems interfering with a child's self-esteem and achievement.) Phoenix, AZ: Sound Listening & Learning Center. www.soundlistening.com/ fchecklist.html.

Tomatis, Alfred A. (1992). *The Conscious Ear.* Rhineback, NY: Station Hill Press.

———, & Billie M. Thompson, trans. (1997). *The Ear and Language.* Ontario, Canada: Stoddart.

ORAL-MOTOR DEVELOPMENT

Frick, Sheila M., Ron Frick, Patricia Oetter, & Eileen W. Richter (1996). *Out of the Mouths of Babes: Discovering the Developmental Significance of the Mouth—a Book Especially for Parents & Other "Grown-ups."* Hugo, MN: PDP Press.

Oetter, Patricia, Eileen W. Richter, & Sheila M. Frick (1995). *M.O.R.E. (Motor, Oral, Respiration, Eyes): Integrating the Mouth with Sensory and Postural Functions* (2nd ed.). Hugo, MN: PDP Press.

SENSORY DIET AND
SENSORY-MOTOR ACTIVITIES

Henry, Diana (1998). *Tool Chest for Teachers, Parents & Students: A Handbook to Facilitate Self-Regulation.* (Accompanies two videos: *Tools for Students: OT Activities for Classroom & Home,* and *Tools for Teachers: an Overview of School Based Occupational Therapy.*) Youngtown, AZ: Henry OT Services.

————, & Tammy Wheeler (2001). *Tools for Parents: A Handbook to Bring Sensory Integration into the Home.* Youngtown, AZ: Henry OT Services.

————, Tammy Wheeler, & Deanna Iris Sava (2004). *Sensory Integration Tools for Teens: Strategies to Promote Sensory Processing.* Youngtown, AZ: Henry OT Services.

Kranowitz, Carol S. (1995). *101 Activities for Kids in Tight Spaces.* New York: St. Martin's.

———— (2002). *Getting Kids in Sync: Sensory-Motor Activities to Help Children Develop Body Awareness & Integrate Their Senses* (video). Las Vegas: Sensory Resources.

———— (2003). *The Out-of-Sync Child Has Fun: Activities for Kids with Sensory Integration Dysfunction.* New York: Perigee.

———— (2004). *The Goodenoughs Get in Sync: A Story for Kids about Sensory Processing Disorder.* Las Vegas: Sensory Resources.

Williams, Mary Sue, & Sherry Shellenberger. *An Introduction to "How Does Your Engine Run?" The Alert Program for Self-Regulation* (1992), and *Take Five! Staying Alert at Home and School* (2002). Albuquerque: TherapyWorks.

Yack, Ellen, Shirley Sutton, & Paula Aquilla (2002). *Building Bridges through Sensory Integration: OT for Children with Autism and other Pervasive Developmental Disorders* (2nd ed.). Las Vegas: Sensory Resources.

SENSORY PROCESSING

Ahn, Roianne, PhD, Lucy Jane Miller, PhD, Sharon Milberger, ScD, & Daniel N. McIntosh, PhD (May/June 2004). Prevalence of parents' perceptions of sensory processing disorders among kindergarten children. *American Journal of Occupational Therapy*, 58(3).

Ayres, A. Jean, PhD (1972). *Sensory Integration and Learning Disorders*. Los Angeles: Western Psychological Services.

——— (1979). *Sensory Integration and the Child*. Los Angeles: Western Psychological Services.

Balzer-Martin, Lynn A., PhD, & C. S. Kranowitz (1992). *The Balzer-Martin Preschool Screening Program Manual*. Washington, DC: St. Columba's.

Bissell, Julie, Jean Fisher, Carol Owens, & Patricia Polcyn (1998). *Sensory Motor Handbook: A Guide for Implementing and Modifying Activities in the Classroom*. San Diego: Academic Press.

Bundy, Anita C., ScD, Shelly J. Lane, PhD, & Elizabeth A. Murray, ScD, eds. (2002). *Sensory Integration: Theory and Practice* (2nd ed.). Philadelphia: F.A. Davis. (I found these chapters particularly helpful: Orchestrating intervention: The art of practice, by Anita C. Bundy, ScD, & Jane A. Koomar, PhD; Visual-spatial abilities, by Anne Henderson, PhD, Charlane Pehoski, ScD, & Elizabeth Murray, ScD; and Sensory modulation; and Structure and function of the sensory systems, both by Shelly J. Lane, Phd.)

Cermak, Sharon, EdD, Alice Miller, Winnie Dunn, PhD, & Occupational Therapy Associates of Watertown (1991). Eastern European adopted children—Developmental and sensory history questionnaire. Boston University.

Dejean, Valerie, & Alex Freer (2002). What is sensory integration? Hand-out from Spectrum Center, Inc., (301) 657-0988 or www.spectrumcenter.com.

Dunn, Winnie, PhD (1997). The impact of sensory processing abilities on the daily lives of young children and their families: A conceptual model. *Infants and Young Children*, 9(4).

————— (1999). *Sensory Profile.* San Antonio: The Psychological Corporation.

————— (2001). The sensations of everyday life: Empirical, theoretical, and pragmatic considerations. The 2001 Eleanor Clarke Slagle Lecture. *American Journal of Occupational Therapy,* 55(6).

Eide, Fernette F., MD (2003). Sensory integration—current concepts and practical implications. *Sensory Integration Special Interest Quarterly,* 26(3). Bethesda, MD: American Occupational Therapy Association (AOTA).

Grooms, Julie (2001). *The Scoop on Sensory Integration: A Resource Created for Teachers and Paraprofessionals.* (16-page booklet.) available from Pocket Full of Therapy, www.pfot.com

Hanft, Barbara E., Lucy Jane Miller, PhD, & Shelly J. Lane, PhD (September 2000). Toward a consensus in terminology in sensory integration theory and practice: Part 3: Observable behaviors: Sensory integration dysfunction. *Sensory Integration Special Interest Section Quarterly,* 23(3). Bethesda, MD: AOTA.

Heller, Sharon, PhD (2002). *Too Loud, Too Bright, Too Fast, Too Tight: What to Do If You Are Sensory Defensive in an Overstimulating World.* New York: HarperCollins.

Kinnealey, Moya, PhD, & Sinclair Smith, ScD (Autumn 2004). A review of research on sensory modulation disorder in adults. *S.I. Focus* magazine.

Koomar, Jane A., PhD, Barbara Friedman, & Elizabeth Woolf, illus. (1998). *The Hidden Senses: Your Muscle Sense* and *The Hidden Senses: Your Balance Sense.* Hugo, MN: PDP Press.

Kranowitz, C.S. (2001). *The Out-of-Sync Child* (video). Las Vegas: Sensory Resources.

Lane, Shelly J., PhD, Lucy Jane Miller, PhD, & Barbara E. Hanft (June 2000). Toward a consensus in terminology in sensory integration theory and practice: Part 2: Sensory integration patterns of function and dysfunction. *Sensory Integration Special Interest Section Quarterly,* 23(2). Bethesda, MD: AOTA.

Mailloux, Zoe (Spring, 1993). The vestibular system: Why is it so critical? *Sensory Integration Quarterly,* 21(1). Torrance, CA: Sensory Integration International.

May-Benson, Teresa A. (December 2000). Creating a consensus on terminology in sensory integration: Comments and reflections. *Sensory Integration Special Interest Section Quarterly,* 23(4). Bethesda, MD: AOTA.

Miller, Lucy Jane, PhD, Sharon A. Cermak, EdD, Shelly J. Lane, PhD, Marie E. Anzalone, ScD, & Jane A. Koomar, PhD (Summer 2004). Position statement on terminology related to sensory integration dysfunction. *S.I. Focus* magazine.

———, & Shelly J. Lane, PhD (March 2000). Toward a consensus in terminology in sensory integration theory and practice: Part 1: Taxonomy of neurophysiological processes. *Sensory Integration Special Interest Section Quarterly,* 23(1). Bethesda, MD: AOTA.

———, with Doris A. Fuller (in press). *Sensational Kids: Hope and Help for Children with Sensory Processing Disorder.* New York: Putnam.

Miller-Kuhaneck, Heather, ed. (2001) *Autism: A Comprehensive Occupational Therapy Approach.* Bethesda, MD: American Occupational Therapy Association. (Particularly helpful chapters include: Alternative and complementary approaches in the treatment of autism, by Patricia S. Lemer; and Sensory integration, by Zoe Mailloux & Susanne Smith Roley.)

Reisman, Judith E. (1997). *Sensory Processing for Parents: From Roots to Wings* (video). University of Minnesota/Fourth Canyon Productions. www.theraproducts.com.

Roley, Susanne Smith, Erna Imperatore Blanche, PhD, & Roseann C. Schaaf, eds. (2001). *Understanding the Nature of Sensory Integration with Diverse Populations.* San Antonio: Therapy Skill Builders. (Particularly helpful chapters include: Proprioception: a cornerstone of sensory integrative intervention, by Erna Imperatore Blanche, PhD, & Roseann C. Schaaf; Clinical applications in sensory modulation

dysfunction: Assessment and intervention considerations,
Lucy Jane Miller, PhD, & Clare Summers; An ecological
model of sensory modulation: Performance of children with
Fragile X syndrome, autistic disorder, attention-
deficit/hyperactivity disorder, and sensory modulation
dysfunction, by Lucy Jane Miller, PhD, Judith E. Reisman,
PhD, Daniel N. McIntosh, PhD, & Jodie Simon, PhD; and
Sensory integration and visual deficits, including blindness, by
Susanne Smith Roley and Colleen Schneck, ScD.)

Smith, Karen A., PhD, & Karen R. Gouze, PhD (2004). *The Sensory-Sensitive Child: Practical Solutions for Out-of-Bounds Behavior*. New York: HarperCollins.

Szklut, Stacey, Sharon Cermak, EdD, Kranowitz, C.S., et al. (1998). *Making Sense of Sensory Integration* (audiotape). Las Vegas: Sensory Resources/Belle Curve.

Trott, Maryann Colby, with Marci K. Laurel & Susan L. Windeck (1993). *SenseAbilities: Understanding Sensory Integration*. Tucson, AZ: Therapy Skill Builders.

Wilbarger, Patricia, & Wilbarger, Julia Leigh (1991). *Sensory Defensiveness in Children Aged 2–12: An Intervention Guide for Parents and Other Caretakers*. Van Nuys, CA: Avanti Educational Programs.

SPECIAL NEEDS

Batshaw, Mark L., MD (2002). *Children with Disabilities: A Medical Primer* (5th ed.). Baltimore: Paul H. Brookes.

DeGangi, Georgia, PhD (2000). *Pediatric Disorders of Regulation in Affect and Behavior: A Therapist's Guide to Assessment and Treatment*. San Diego: Academic Press.

Greene, Ross W., PhD (2001). *The Explosive Child: A New Approach for Understanding and Parenting Easily Frustrated, Chronically Inflexible Children* (2nd ed.). New York: HarperCollins.

Greenspan, Stanley I., MD, Chair (1994). *Diagnostic Classification (of Mental Health and Developmental Disorders of Infancy and Early Childhood): 0–3.* Arlington, VA: Zero to Three, National Center for Clinical Infant Programs.

——— (1995). *The Challenging Child: Understanding, Raising, and Enjoying the Five "Difficult" Types of Children.* Reading, MA: Addison-Wesley.

———, & Serena Wieder, with Robin Simons (1998). *The Child with Special Needs: Encouraging Intellectual and Emotional Growth.* Reading, MA: Perseus.

Klass, Perri, MD, & Eileen Costello, MD (2003). *Quirky Kids: Understanding and Helping Your Child Who Doesn't Fit In—When to Worry and When Not to Worry.* New York: Ballantine.

Kurcinka, Mary Sheedy (1992). *Raising Your Spirited Child: A Guide for Parents Whose Child is More Intense, Sensitive, Perceptive, Persistent, Energetic.* New York: HarperCollins.

Lemer, Patricia S. (1995). Attention deficits: A developmental approach. (Brochure.) Santa Ana, CA: Optometric Extension Program.

Papolos, Demitri F., MD, & Janice Papolos (1999). *The Bipolar Child: The Definitive and Reassuring Guide to Childhood's Most Misunderstood Disorder.* New York: Broadway.

Rapp, Doris, MD (1992). *Is This Your Child? Discovering and Treating Unrecognized Allergies.* New York: Perennial Currents.

Quick Reference to the Diagnostic Criteria from DSM-IV (1994). Washington, DC: American Psychiatric Association.

Silver, Larry B. (1999). *Dr. Larry Silver's Advice to Parents on ADHD* (2nd ed.). New York: Three Rivers Press.

Turecki, Stanley, MD, with Leslie Tonner (2000). *The Difficult Child* (2nd ed.). New York: Bantam.

Zero to Three (1994). *Diagnostic Classification of Mental Health and Developmental Disorders of Infancy and Early Childhood.* Arlington, VA: National Center for Clinical Infant Programs.

Speech, Language, and Communication

Agin, Marilyn C., MD, Lisa F. Geng, & Malcolm J. Nicholl (2003). *The Late Talker: What to Do if Your Child Isn't Talking Yet.* New York: St. Martin's.

Kashman, Nancy, & Janet Mora (2002). *The Sensory Connection: An OT and SLP Team Approach.* Las Vegas: Sensory Resources.

Mehrabian, Albert, PhD (1968). Communication without words. *Psychology Today,* 2(4).

Nowicki, Stephen, Jr., PhD, & Marshall P. Duke, PhD (1992). *Helping the Child Who Doesn't Fit In.* Atlanta: Peachtree.

————, & Elisabeth A. Martin (1996). *Teaching Your Child the Language of Social Success.* Atlanta: Peachtree.

Whitney, Rondalyn Varney (2002). *Bridging the Gap: Raising a Child with Nonverbal Learning Disorder.* New York: Perigee.

Vision

Barber, Anne R., OD, ed. (1999). *Behavioral Aspects of Vision Care: Vision and Sensory Integration,* 40(2). Santa Ana, CA: Optometric Extension Program Foundation. (Particularly pertinent articles include: Sensory integration and vision, by Sharon Berger, OD; and The neurofunctional basis of sensorimotor integration: integrating vision with the other senses, by Merrill D. Bowan, OD.)

Brockett, Sally (Summer 1995). Vision therapy: A beneficial intervention for developmental disabilities. *New Developments,* 1(2). Bethesda, MD: Developmental Delay Resources (DDR).

Cirigliano, Suzette (August 2004). About vision problems. www.Vision-Therapy.com

———— (October 2004). Visual abilities, vision therapy, and the myths of 20/20 vision. www.vision-therapycom/drtoler/booklet.htm

Gould, Marge Christensen, & Herman Gould, OD (December 2003). A clear vision for equity and opportunity. *Phi Delta Kappan, The Professional Journal for Education,* 85(4). (About undetected and uncorrected visual problems.)

Hickman, Lois, & Rebecca Hutchins, OD (2000). *Seeing Clearly: Fun Activities for Improving Visual Skills.* Las Vegas: Sensory Resources.

Kavner, Richard S., OD (1985). *Your Child's Vision: A Parent's Guide to Seeing, Growing, and Developing.* New York: Simon and Schuster.

Lane, Kenneth A., (1993). *Developing Your Child for Success: Easy to Follow Activities to Develop Children's Perceptual and Motor Skills and Prepare Them for Their Early School Years.* Lewisville, TX: Learning Potentials.

Optometric Extension Program Foundation, Inc. (undated). *Vision Checklists* (to help parents identify behavioral signs of visual problems caused by vestibular dysfunction). Santa Ana, CA: www.oep.org

Shidlofsky, Charles, OD (Winter 2003). Visual processing and perception: A piece of the puzzle. Dallas: *S.I. Challenge* newsletter.

RELATED READING

Brazelton, T. Berry, MD, & Stanley I. Greenspan, MD (2000). *The Irreducible Needs of Children: What Every Child Must Have to Grow, Learn, and Flourish.* New York: Perseus.

Greenspan, Stanley I., MD, with Jacqueline Salmon (1993). *Playground Politics: Understanding the Emotional Life of Your School-Age Child.* Reading, MA: Addison-Wesley.

Rubin, Kenneth H., PhD, with Andrea Thompson (2002). *The Friendship Factor: Helping Our Children Navigate Their Social World—and Why It Matters for Their Success and Happiness.* New York: Viking.

INDEX

Academic learning
    problems with, 28, 98
    and sensory processing, 11, 67, 97 98,
        302–303
Activities, sensory motor
    active v. passive, 6, 256
    for auditory sense, 236–237
    in occupational therapy, 220–221,
        229–230
    at school, xxi, 4, 6, 256
    for proprioceptive sense, 229–230
    for self-help skills, 240–243
    in sensory diet, 228–231
    for sensory motor skills, 238–240
    for tactile sense, 231–233
    for vestibular sense, 233–235
    for visual sense, 237
Activity level
    in ADHD, 29
    development of, 301
    screening for, 41, 45
    and SPD, 8–9, 23, 26–27
    treatment for, 224, 231, 263
Adaptive behavior/responses, 11, 48, 56,
    63, 69
Allergies, 21, 36–37

Anzalone, Marie, ScD, 10
Aquilla, Paula, 229
Arousal level, 23, 26–27, 138,
    149
Asperger syndrome, 33, 39
Associated problems
    allergies, 36–37
    arousal, activity level, and attention, 23,
        26–27
    Asperger Syndrome, 33, 39
    attachment, 28, 99
    Attention Deficit/Hyperactivity
        Disorder, 21–22, 29–30, 39
    autism, 31–33
    bipolar disorder, 34
    digestion/elimination, 25–26
    digestion/nutrition, 24–26, 224
    dyslexia, 31
    eating, 24–25
    genetic syndromes, 35–36
    learning disabilities, 22, 30–31
    neurological disabilities, 22
    Nonverbal Learning Disorder (NLD),
        33–34
    Obsessive Compulsive Disorder (OCD),
        34

Associated problems (*continued*)
    Pervasive Developmental Disorder
        (PDD), 31–33, 39
    psychological problems, 34
    selective mutism, 35
    self-regulation, 23
    sleeping, 23–24
    social/emotional problems, 27–28
Attachment, 28, 99, 105, 300
Attention
    and auditory sense, 18, 178–179, 181,
        185–188
    and autism, 31
    problems with, xxii, 9, 21, 26–27, 35,
        46, 69–70, 73–75
    and proprioceptive sense, 7, 208–209
    and sensory processing, 55, 57–59, 61,
        64, 67, 69, 287, 290, 301–302
    and tactile sense, 4, 81–82, 84, 87–88,
        103, 157, 251
    treatment for, 218, 253, 256, 258, 260
    and vestibular sense, 117, 122, 207–208,
        234
    and visual sense, 16, 153–154, 157–158,
        160, 162, 164, 166, 172, 252
Attention Deficit/Hyperactivity Disorder
    (ADHD), 21–22, 29–30, 39, 194–195
Auditory dysfunction
    and autism, 182
    case example, 174–176
    checklists, 16, 18, 44, 186–190
    discrimination problems, 18, 21,
        183–185, 187
    modulation problems, 181–183, 186–187
    overresponsivity/auditory defensiveness,
        70, 181–182, 186–187
    sensory seeking, 183
    speech/language problems, 179–180,
        184–185, 188–189
    treatment for, 184–185, 223
    underresponsivity, 182–183
Auditory sense
    defensive/discriminative components,
        177–180
    development of, 176, 299–302
    functions of, 176–180
    integration with vestibular and other
        senses, 157, 177
    sensory-motor activities for, 236–237
    speech and language, 179–180
Auditory training, 185, 223

Autism
    and auditory dysfunction, 181–182
    on SI Continuum, 38–39
    with SPD, 21–22, 31–33
    and visual dysfunction, 162–163
Autistic Spectrum Disorder (ASD), 32
Aversive response, 71
Ayres, A. Jean, PhD
    on dyspraxia, 77
    four levels of sensory development,
        66–68, 299–303
    on parenting, 263
    on postural responses, 61, 76
    on prevalence of sensory problems, 39
    research, xiv, 38
    on sensory input, 55–56
    Sensory Integration and the Child, xxiii,
        115
    SI theory/concepts, xiv, ix, xxiii, 9–10,
        113–115, 221
    SI therapy, xv, xxiii, 221
    on touch, 83
    on vision, 162

Balance
    and auditory sense, 177, 180, 185
    problems with, 15, 17, 19, 276, 286
    and proprioceptive sense, 6, 151
    and sensory processing, 290, 296–297
    treatment for, 218, 220, 223–224, 234,
        268, 279
    and vestibular sense, 26, 78, 113–116,
        123, 131–133, 205, 207–208
    and visual sense, 157, 160, 167, 173
Balzer-Martin, Lynn, PhD, xxiii–xxv
Behavior
    adaptive, 63
    adult's response, 259–260, 263–265
    attachment, 28, 99
    and auditory sense, 174 ff.
    and proprioceptive sense, 134 ff.
    and vestibular sense, 110 ff.
    and visual sense, 152 ff.
Berard, Guy, MD, 185, 223
Bilateral coordination
    and auditory sense, 177, 185
    development of, 300–301
    and postural responses, 19, 61, 76
    treatment for, 218, 221, 238–240, 242
    and vestibular sense, 112, 125–126,
        131–133

Binocularity, 76, 158, 161, 301. *See also*
  Visual sense
Bipolar disorder, 34
Birth trauma, 37
Body awareness (Body percept, Body
  scheme)
  development of, 300
  and proprioceptive sense, 135, 140, 144,
    150
  with Sensory Discrimination Disorder,
    17, 75
  and tactile sense, 91–92, 107
  and vestibular sense, 127, 132
Body position. *See* Proprioceptive
  dysfunction
Brain. *See also* Central nervous system
  brain-behavior connection, xiv, 11–12
  parts, 289–295
  CNS processing in, 55–68, 289–297
  evolution of, 283–284, 288–289
  "indigestion" of, 69
  triune, 288–289
Bundy, Anita, PhD, 63

Causes of SPD, 37–38
Central nervous system (CNS)
  auditory processing in, 176
  development of, 66–68, 283 ff.
  discrimination in, 59–61, 74–75
  excitation and inhibition in, 57, 59,
    69–70
  habituation in, 58–59
  integration in, 56–57
  modulation in, 57–59, 69–74
  plasticity in, 48
  proprioceptive processing in, 137, 139
  reception and detection in, 56
  and sensory-based motor
    skills/disorders, 61–62, 75–77
  sensory processing in, 11, 55–68, 79,
    137, 284–297
  reception/detection in, 56
  SPD in, xxiii, 11, 69, 79 (chart)
  tactile processing in, 83–90
  vestibular processing in, 113, 115, 123,
    127
  vision processing in, 155–156
Cermak, Sharon, EdD, 10, 41
Chiropractic, 223
Classroom strategies, 251–260
Communication, 28–35, 98, 166

Coordination problems. *See* Bilateral
  coordination
Coping skills, 261–272
Craniosacral therapy, 223
Crossing the midline, 19, 76, 125, 133,
  239, 301

Defensive/discriminative components, 52,
  59–61, 70
  in autism, 32
  in auditory sense, 67, 70, 177–181, 216
  in tactile sense, 24, 70, 83–86, 89–90,
    100–103, 196, 201
  treatment for, 216, 220, 243, 258
  in vestibular sense, 115
  in visual sense, 67, 157–166
Development of sensory processing,
  66–68, 299–303
Developmental delays, 38, 47
Diagnosis, 193–216
  auditory dysfunction, 44, 186–190
  screenings/evaluations, xvi, 40–47,
    193–195, 212–219
  caveats, 77–78
  information sources, 212–214
  mistaken, xxiv, 21, 195
  and parental documentation, 198–199,
    226
  parental emotions about, 193–198
  proprioceptive dysfunction, 148–151
  Sensory-Motor History Questionnaire,
    41–47
  tactile dysfunction, 41–43, 101–109
  taste and smell dysfunction, 45
  vestibular dysfunction, 43–44,
    129–133
  visual dysfunction, 44, 169–173
Diagnostic and Statistical Manual (DSM),
  217
*Diagnostic Classification of Mental Health
  and Developmental Disorders of Infancy
  and Early Childhood*, 217
Discipline, 265–266
Digestion/Elimination, 25–26, 53, 132
Digestion/Nutrition, 21, 23–25, 36, 224
Documentation by parents, 198–212, 226
Dorfman, Kelly, 38–39
Down syndrome, 35, 163
Dunn, Winnie, PhD, 41
Dysfunction in Sensory Integration (DSI), 9
Dyslexia, 18, 31, 126

Dyspraxia/Praxis
  case examples, 6–7, 110–112, 134–136, 152–154, 209–210
  checklists for, 20, 108–109, 133, 150
  and proprioceptive sense, 139, 147, 150
  as a Sensory-Based Motor Disorder, 19–20, 77, 245
  and tactile sense, 95, 108–109
  and vestibular sense, 112, 126–128, 133
  and visual sense, 154, 167–168

Early intervention, xxv, 47–48. *See also* Treatment/therapy
Eating/feeding
  and discrimination disorder, 17
  examples of problems with, 200–204, 208–209, 215
  and fine motor skills, 17, 20, 94, 108, 132, 161
  and genetic syndromes, 35
  improving, 241–242
  and regulatory disorders, 24–25
  screening for, 45–46
  sensory processing for, 52, 299
  and sensory modulation disorders, 16, 70–73
Emotional security
  proprioceptive sense for, 148, 151
  tactile sense for, 98–100, 102
  vestibular sense for, 128, 133
Emotional skills
  checklists for, 47, 102, 129–130, 133, 151
  development of, xxiv, 34, 299 ff.
  do's and don'ts for coping, 267–272
  and gravitational insecurity, 119–120
  parenting techniques for, 263–267
  in regulatory disorders, 27–29
  related to SPD, 21, 34
  treatment for, 49, 219, 225
Evaluation. *See* Diagnosis
Eye-hand coordination
  problems with, 20, 108, 167, 172
  development of, 67, 160, 302
  treatment for, 169, 222, 238
Eye movement. *See* Visual sense

Fetal alcohol syndrome, 35–36
Fight/fight/freeze/fright response, 71, 52, 277, 288–289
  and auditory dysfunction, 181
  and tactile dysfunction, 14, 85, 102

  and vestibular dysfunction, 113, 119
  and visual dysfunction, 162
Fine motor and gross motor control
  development of, 290, 303
  and dyspraxia, xiv, 20, 108
  and proprioceptive sense, 139, 145
  sensory activities for, 218, 221, 224, 238, 242, 258
  and tactile sense, 94–95, 108
  and vestibular sense, 132
  and visual sense, 160–161, 173
Floortime, 263
Fragile X syndrome, 35
Frick, Sheila, 223

Gender, 35, 39
Genetic predisposition to SPD, 37
Grading of movement, 12, 17, 145–146, 150–151
Grandin, Temple, PhD, 32–33
Gravitational insecurity
  treatment for, 221, 233
  and vestibular overresponsivity, 112, 117, 119–120, 129–130
Gravity, 114
Greenspan, Stanley, MD, 10, 263, 273
Gross motor control. *See* Fine motor control
Gustatory sense, 53, 65. *See also* Taste

Habituation, 29, 58
Hand preference, 19, 67, 125, 132, 301
Hearing. *See* Auditory sense
Heavy work activity, 6, 142
Hippotherapy, 224
Home activities for sensory processing, 231–243
Home schooling, 250
Hyperactivity, xxiv, 21, 29, 36
Hypersensitivity, 70. *See also* Sensory overresponsivity
Hyposensitivity, 72. *See also* Sensory underresponsivity

Impulsivity, 27, 29, 45, 87, 112
Individuals with Disabilities Education Improvement Act of 2004 (IDEA 04), 213–214, 217
Inclusion, xxiii
Individualized Education Program (IEP), 250

Infancy
  and SPD, 4, 102, 120
  typical, 60, 66, 82, 84, 98, 115, 157, 286, 299
Inhibition, 57, 59, 69–70
Institutionalization, 37
Insurance coverage, 9, 217–218
Interoception, 26, 54
Intersensory integration, 51
Intervention. *See* Treatment/Therapy
Intolerance to movement, 112, 117–118, 129

Kinesthesia, 31, 137
Koomar, Jane, PhD, 63
Kurcinka, Mary, 263

Lane, Shelly, PhD, 10
Language disabilities, xiii–xvii. *See also* Speech/Language
Learned helplessness, 268
Learning
  active v. passive, 256
  and tactile sense, 97–98
  types of, 11–12
Learning disabilities, xiii–xvii, 21–22, 30–31
Look-alike symptoms, 21

MacLean, Paul, MD, 288
Maddux Foundation, xxiv
Martial arts, 224
Mental health, 21, 29–35
  and OT, 219
  problems, secondary to SPD, xv
  professionals, xv, xxiv
Mental retardation, 35, 213
Miller, Lucy Jane, PhD, ix–xi, 10–11, 29
Modulation. *See* Sensory modulation
Motor control/Motor coordination
  and auditory sense, 179–180, 185, 223
  development of, 289, 301
  problems with, xvi, 20, 30, 262
  and proprioceptive sense, 138–139, 145, 150, 303
  and tactile sense, 93–95, 108
  treatment for, 221–223, 234, 240
  and vestibular sense, 122, 205
  and visual sense, 169, 222
Motor planning. *See* Praxis

Movement
  active and passive, 6, 140, 205, 220
  and auditory sense, 176, 184–186, 189–190
  and dyspraxia, 77, 92, 108, 112, 246
  as basis of learning, 156
  checklists for problems, 15, 17–19, 43–44
  increased tolerance for, 112, 121, 130, 204–205
  intolerance to, 112, 129, 276, 281
  linear and rotary, 113–114, 116, 118, 121, 206, 233
  and non-SPD problems, 23, 26, 31–32, 35–36
  and sensory discrimination disorder, 17, 75, 150, 176
  and sensory modulation disorders, 71–74
  and postural disorder, 75
  and proprioceptive sense, 54, 136 ff., 150, 208–209
  skills, development of, 11, 299–301
  and smooth sensory processing, xxi, 51, 57, 61, 64, 67, 283, 290–291, 293
  and SPD, xiv, 11, 69, 76
  and tactile sense, 82, 92–95, 104, 106, 108
  treatment to improve, 220–224, 230–231, 233, 256, 268
  and vestibular sense, 5–6, 54, 112 ff., 204–206
  and visual sense, 154–161, 163, 165–173
Movement breaks, in classroom, 256
Muscle control, 15, 17, 35
Muscle tone
  problems with, 19, 25–26, 75, 124–125, 131, 149, 205–206, 273
  treatment for, 224
  typically developing, 61, 78, 113, 124, 290, 300

Nervous system. *See also* Central nervous system
  and allergies, 36
  autonomic, 284
  central, 48, 56–57, 64, 70, 74, 79
  peripheral, 56, 64, 284, 288, 294–295
  and eating problems, 25
  and SPD, xiv, xxiii–xxiv, 70, 74, 79
  and typical sensory processing, 283 ff.

Nervous system (*continued*)
  treatment for, 48, 195, 220–224, 228–230
Neurologist, 221
Nonverbal learning disorder, 33–34
Nutrition, 21, 23, 25–26, 224

Obsessive compulsive disorder, 34
Ocular control, 76, 221. *See also* Visual sense
Occupational therapy (OT)
  activities in, 220–221, 229–231
  for problems associated with SPD, 26, 29, 36
  evaluation of SPD, 40, 215–219
  health professionals, 214, 219–220
  using sensory integration framework (OT/SI), ix–x, 36, 47, 193, 195
  research, 38
  at school, 31, 217, 259
  sensory diet, 23, 49, 212, 227 ff., 279
  for SPD, ix–x, xxv, 9, 29, 38–39, 47–49, 220–222, 225–226
  for vestibular and auditory senses, 185
  for visual sense, 169
Occupational Therapy Associates-Watertown, 41
Olfactory sense, 53, 253, 291 *See also* Smell
Optometry and visual therapy, 169, 215, 222
Oral-motor problems
  and dyspraxia, 20
  and eating, 24
  and speech, 97
  treatment for, 25, 222, 232
Osten, Beth, 10

Parents
  advice for, 263–272
  advocating for child, 245, 247–249, 267
  comments from, 193–195, 247, 261–262, 273–274, 279–281
  communicating with teachers, 244–250
  support for, 212–214
  understanding effects of SPD, 245–247, 273–279
Penfield, Wilder, 294
Perceptual motor skills, 67, 224, 301–302
Pervasive developmental disorder, 32
Physical therapy, xxv, 31, 36, 217, 222

Picky eating, 24, 141, 149
Postural control/Postural responses
  and auditory sense, 180
  as end result of sensory processing, 56, 61–62, 300–301
  and vestibular sense, 114
  and visual sense, 156–157, 160
Postural disorder. *See also* Dyspraxia
  and auditory sense, 185, 223
  checklists for, 18–19, 131–133
  and ocular control, 76
  and proprioceptive sense, 6, 140–141, 146–147, 151, 210–211
  sensory slumper, 75–76
  and toileting, 26
  treatment for, 49, 216, 218, 220, 223–224, 234, 253
  and vestibular sense, 112, 116, 123–125, 131, 205–206
  and visual sense, 162–163, 168–169, 173
Praxis (Motor planning). *See also* Dyspraxia
  development of, 301
  as end result of sensory processing, 62
  for fine and gross motor control, 20, 93–95, 139, 145
  ideation, 62
  perceptual motor therapy for, 224
  and proprioceptive sense, 136, 139, 144, 146, 148
  as sensory-based motor skill, 19–20, 61–62, 77
  and tactile sense, 92–93
  and vestibular sense, 126–127
Prematurity, 37
Prenatal/postnatal circumstances, 37
Proprioceptive dysfunction
  and body awareness, 135, 139–141, 144
  and body position, 15, 17, 19, 91, 139, 150
  case examples, 6–7, 134–136
  checklists, 15, 17, 148–151
  and digestion/elimination, 26
  and emotional security, 148, 151
  and grading of movement, 145–146, 150
  and motor control, 145
  overresponsivity, 140–141, 149
  parental documentation, example, 208–212
  and postural stability, 140–141, 146–147, 151

and praxis/dyspraxia, 136, 139, 141, 144, 146–148, 150
sensory seeking, 142–143, 149
underresponsivity, 141–142, 149
and visual processing, 156–157
Proprioceptive sense
development of, 299–301, 303
functions of, 54, 68, 136–139
integration with other senses, 91, 93, 137–138, 156, 179
sensory-motor activities for, 142, 235–236
Psychotherapy, 225

Rainy Day Indoor Playground, 247
Rapp, Doris, MD, 36
Reading, 7, 11, 31
Record keeping/documentation, 198 ff, 226
Regulatory disorders
arousal/activity level/attention, 26–27
digestion/elimination, 25–26
eating, 24–25
self-regulation, 23
sleeping, 23–24
social/emotional functioning, 27–29
Research, 29, 38
Rogers, Carl, PhD, 259

St. Columba's Nursery School, xxi, 49, 227, 246, 280–281
School
classroom strategies, 251–260
difficulties for child with SPD, 245–247
homeschooling, 250
home-school partnership, 244–249
public v. private, 250
special education, 213, 250
Screening. *See* Diagnosis
Section 504, *Rehabilitation Act of* 1973, 214
Selective mutism, 35
Self-esteem
problems with, xxiv, 28, 117, 128, 133, 173, 190, 198, 210, 277
sensory processing for, 67, 177, 302
treatment for, 49, 185, 211, 219, 223, 261, 268
Self-help skills (bathing, dressing, feeding, sleeping, handling objects)
development of, 62–63, 301
improving, 23–24, 48–50, 220, 222, 236, 240–243, 268

and proprioceptive sense, 139–141, 148, 150
and SPD, 23–28, 275
screening for, 41, 45–46
and tactile sense, 4, 85–86, 91, 94, 104, 200–203, 278, 280
and vestibular sense, 127, 131
and visual sense, 161, 172
Self therapy, 116, 184, 206, 268
Senses. *See also* Auditory sense, Proprioceptive sense, Tactile sense, Vestibular sense, and Visual sense
external (environmental, or far), 51–54
exteroception, 52
gustatory, 53, 65
internal (body-centered), 53–54
interoception, 55
olfactory, 53
Sensitization, 58
Sensory Based Motor Skills
problems with, 13, 18–20
as end result of sensory processing, 61
motor learning, 11
postural responses, 61–62
praxis, 62–63
Sensory Based Motor Disorder
case examples, 110–112
checklist for, 18–20
classification of, 10
definition of, 75–77
Dyspraxia, 19–20, 77
Postural Disorder, 18–19, 75–77
Sensory craver, 73
Sensory defensiveness, 70
Sensory diet. *See* Occupational therapy
Sensory discrimination
precedence over sensory defensiveness (chart), 60
process, 59–61
Sensory Discrimination Disorder
auditory, 18, 174–176
checklist for, 13, 17–18
classification of, 10
definition of, 17–18, 74–75
proprioceptive, 17, 150
tactile, 17, 89–90
vestibular, 17
visual, 18, 152–154
Sensory fluctuator, 74, 89
Sensory fumbler, 77

Sensory integration
    four levels of sensory integration, 67,
        299–303
    dysfunction of, xxiii, 9
    theory of, ix
Sensory Integration (SI) Continuum,
    38–39
Sensory Integration Dysfunction (DSI),
    xxiii, 9
Sensory Integration (SI) therapy, ix, xv,
    xxv–xxvi, 23–25, 33–34, 39, 195
Sensory jumbler, 74–75
Sensory modulation, 57–59
Sensory Modulation Disorder (SMD)
    in auditory sense, 181–184, 186–187
    classification, 10
    fluctuation, 74, 89
    gravitational insecurity, 119–120
    overresponsivity, 14–16, 70–72, 85–86
    in proprioceptive sense, 140–143,
        149–150
    sensory seeking, 8, 14–16, 73–74, 87–88
    symptoms, 13–16
    in tactile sense, 85–90, 102–107
    underresponsivity, 14–16, 72–73, 87,
        120–121
    in vestibular sense, 117–122, 129–131
    in visual sense, 163–165, 170–171
Sensory Motor History Questionnaire,
    40–47
Sensory motor skills (*See also* Sensory
    Based Motor Skills)
    activities to promote self help skills,
        240–243
    activities to promote sensory processing,
        231–243
    and adaptive behavior, 63
    for bilateral coordination, 239–240
    intervention for, xxv
    questionnaire for, 40–45
    in Sensory Based Motor Disorder, 19–20
Sensory overresponsivity. (*See* Sensory
    Modulation Disorder)
Sensory processing. *See also* Sensory
    Processing Disorder.
    comparison to SPD (chart), 79
    components of, 55–64
    defensiveness, 60–61
    definition of, 55
    development of, 66–68
    discrimination, 59–60

integration, 56–57
internal/external, 52–55
modulation, 57–59
reception and detection, 56
Sensory Processing Disorder (SPD)
    with ADHD, 21, 29–30
    with allergies, 36–37
    with Asperger syndrome, 33
    in auditory sense, 180, ff.
    with autism, 21–22, 31–33
    with bipolar disorder, 34
    case examples, 4–8
    categories and subtypes, 10
    causes, 37–38
    common symptoms, 13–20
    definition/explanation of, ix, xxvi, 9, 68
        ff.
    diagnosis of, 212–216
    with dyslexia, 31
    gender, 39
    with genetic syndromes, 35–36
    identification of, xxiv, 3, 21, 41–47,
        77–79, 195–199
    intervention of, xxv, 47–48, 195–197
    with learning disability, 30–31
    with nonverbal learning disorder, 33–34
    with obsessive compulsive disorder, 34
    prevalence of, 39
    in proprioceptive sense, 139 ff.
    with psychological problems, 34
    with regulatory disorder, 23–29
    research in, 29, 38
    with selective mutism, 35
    in tactile sense, 84 ff.
    in vestibular sense, 116 ff.
    in visual sense, 162 ff.
Sensory Processing Machine, 283–197
Sensory seeking. *See also* Sensory
    Modulation Disorder
    auditory, 183
    case example, 7–8
    proprioceptive, 142–143, 149
    sensory craver, 73
    as Sensory Modulation Disorder, 73–74
    tactile, 87–88, 106–107
    vestibular, 121–122, 130–131
    visual, 164–165
Sensory slumper, 75
Sensory underresponsivity
    auditory, 182–183
    proprioceptive, 141–142, 149

sensory disregarder, 72–73
in Sensory Modulation Disorder, 14–16, 72–73, 87
tactile, 105–106
vestibular, 120–122, 130
visual, 154, 164
Silver, Larry B., MD, xiii–xvii, 224
Six caveats, 77–78
Sleeping. *See* Self help skills
Smell
problems with, 16, 18, 24, 45, 253
and sensory processing, 53, 155, 157, 286, 289, 291, 296
Social skills. *See also* Emotional skills
attachment, 28, 99
and auditory sense, 181, 185
and autism, 32
communication, 28, 35, 98, 166
and gravitational insecurity, 119–120
interactions with others, xiv, 13, 49, 68–70, 75, 246, 250
and proprioceptive sense, 17
and regulatory disorders, 27–29
screening for, 47
and tactile sense, 100–101, 105
treatment for, 48–49
and visual sense, 18, 166
Speech/language
and auditory sense, 177, 179–181, 183–185, 188–190
development of, 286, 289, 292–293, 295, 302
expressive/receptive language, 179–180, 184, 188–189
promoting at home and school, 206, 236, 255, 263
problems associated with SPD, xiv, 16, 20–21, 28, 30–36, 71–73
and proprioceptive sense, 179
and tactile sense, 83, 94, 96–97, 108, 179
and vestibular sense, 112, 117, 179, 276
and visual sense, 160, 167
treatment for, xv, xxv, 184–185, 213, 215, 217, 218, 222–224
Special education, 213, 250
Special needs
children with, xxii–xxiii
in school/classroom, 246–249, 258–259
Stretch, 82, 137
Sutton, Shirley, 229
Syndromes, genetic, 35–36

Tactile defensiveness, 70
Tactile discrimination disorder, 89–90, 107–108
Tactile dysfunction
and academic learning, 97–98
and body awareness, 91–92
case examples, 4–5, 8, 80–82
checklists, 14, 17, 41–43, 101–109
and eating, 24
and emotional security, 98–100
and fine motor control, 94–95
and gross motor control, 93–94
and language, 96–97
parental documentation, example, 199–204
and praxis (motor planning) and dyspraxia, 92–94, 108–109
overresponsivity, 24, 85–87, 102–105
poor discrimination, 89–90, 107–108
sensory combination, 89
sensory seeking, 87–88, 106–107
and social skills, 100–101
and toileting, 26
underresponsivity, 26, 87, 105–106
and visual discrimination, 95–96
Tactile sense
defensive/discriminative components, 83–86, 89–90
functions of, 68, 82–84
integration with other senses, 91, 93, 95–96, 137, 157, 179
sensory-motor activities for, 231–233
Taste
problems with, 16, 18, 24–25, 45, 58
and sensory processing, 52–53, 65, 157, 289
Tomatis, Alfred, MD, 185, 223
Treatment/Therapy. *See also* Sensory Integration Therapy
for ADHD vs. treatment for SPD, 29
auditory training, 185, 223
chiropractic, 223
craniosacral therapy, 223
hippotherapy, 224
intervention for, xv, xxv, 195–197
martial arts, 224
nutritional, 36–37, 224
occupational therapy using sensory integration, 195, 219–221, 225–226
payment for, 217–218
perceptual motor, 224

Treatment/Therapy (*continued*)
  physical therapy, 222
  psychotherapy, 225
  parental documentation, 226
  of SPD, xxv–xxvi, 4, 23–24, 47–49,
    219–226
  speech/language, 184–185, 222
  support for, 212–214
  types of, 221–222
  vision therapy, 222–223
Tribune brain, 288–289
Trott, Maryann Colby, 263
Turecki, Stanley, M.D., 263

Underconnectivity theory, 31
Unilateral coordination, 19
Upledger, John, D.O., 223

Vestibular dysfunction
  and attention, 122
  and auditory processing, 126, 184–186
  and behavior, 117
  and bilateral coordination, 125–126,
    131–133
  case examples, 5–6, 110–112
  checklists, 15, 17, 43–44, 129–133
  and emotional security, 128, 133
  and gravitational insecurity, 119–120,
    129–130
  intolerance to movement, 117–118, 129
  and language, 117, 184–185
  and movement and balance, 116, 118,
    123, 130–131
  and muscle tone, 124–125, 131–133
  overresponsivity, 117–118
  parental documentation, example,
    204–208
  and postural responses, 112, 116
  and praxis (motor planning) and
    dyspraxia, 112, 126–128, 133
  sensory seeking/increased tolerance for
    movement, 121–122, 130–131
  underresponsivity, 120–121, 130
  and visual processing, 117, 126, 156–157
Vestibular sense
  development of, 115–116, 299–301
  evolution of, 114–115
  functions of, 54, 68, 113–116
  integration with other senses, 137–138,
    177, 179
  sensory-motor activities for, 233–235
Vibration, 82, 106, 114
Vision therapy, 222
Visual dysfunction (Poor binocularity, Poor
  ocular-control)
  and autism, 162
  and basic visual skills, 169–170
  case examples, 152–154, 205–206
  checklists, 15, 18, 44, 169–173
  discrimination problems, 18, 21,
    162–163, 165–166, 171–172
  overresponsivity/visual defensiveness,
    154, 163–164, 170–171
  and postural responses, 76, 168–169
  sensory seeking, 164–165
  treatment for, 159, 216, 221–222, 224
  underresponsivity, 154, 164, 170–171
  and vestibular sense, 116–117
  visual dyspraxia/poor visual-motor
    skills, 154, 166–168, 172–173
Visual sense
  basic visual skills, 158–159, 169–170
  binocularity, 158, 161, 301
  defensive/discriminative components,
    157–162, 165–166, 171–172
  development, 300–303
  discrimination, 95–96, 159–160
  eye movement/ocular control, 156, 158,
    161, 300–301
  and eyesight, 155–156
  functions, of, 155–157, 161–162
  integration with other senses, 95–96,
    138, 156–157
  interesting facts about, 156
  sensory-motor activities for, 237
  therapy for, 222
  visual-motor skills, 160–162,
    166–168

Wilbarger, Patricia, and Julia Wilbarger,
  PhD, 229
Writing, 214, 258

Yack, Ellen, 229